Praise for
Feeding the Hungry Ghost by Ellen Kanner

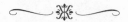

"Just what it takes, on and off the plate, to enjoy a richer life today."
— Mireille Guiliano, author of *French Women Don't Get Fat*

"Beyond being a collection of recipes, this is a book about living. Ellen is like having an elfin, white, Jewish, vegan Oprah whispering in your ear that 'it's going to be more than okay, honey — it's going to be magical!'"
— from the foreword by Norman Van Aken, coauthor (with Justin Van Aken) of *My Key West Kitchen*

FEEDING *the* HUNGRY GHOST

FEEDING *the* HUNGRY GHOST

LIFE, FAITH, *and* WHAT TO EAT FOR DINNER

ELLEN KANNER

Foreword by Norman Van Aken

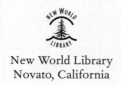

New World Library
Novato, California

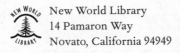 New World Library
14 Pamaron Way
Novato, California 94949

Earlier versions of some content were originally published in the *Huffington Post*, the *Miami Herald*, and *Culinate*.

Text design by Tona Pearce Myers

Library of Congress Cataloging-in-Publication Data is available.

First printing, February 2013
ISBN 978-1-60868-164-8
Printed in the USA on 100% postconsumer-waste recycled paper

 New World Library is proud to be a Gold Certified Environmentally Responsible Publisher. Publisher certification awarded by Green Press Initiative. www.greenpressinitiative.org

10 9 8 7 6 5 4 3 2 1

For Lewis and Marcia Kanner,
the best omnivorous parents a vegan girl could have.
Thanks for always having faith in me.

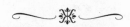

CONTENTS

CHAPTER 2. THE FLOWERING   51

CHAPTER 3. THE HARVEST 105

CHAPTER 4. THE COMPOST 161

FOREWORD

I have favorite quotes from this book already. But before I share a couple, let me harken back. When I was much younger, I'd buy albums at the music store. Now that I have carbon-dated myself, let me say *why* I'm thinking this way in regard to *Feeding the Hungry Ghost* by Ellen Kanner. There were albums that you would put on the turntable and after two listens you would get a kind of *glow*, and that glow was due to the fact that you knew deep inside that this album was going to reveal more and more gems with each listening. Here's one from Ellen that I underlined immediately in my copy of this beautiful new book:

> *"Prayer is attentiveness — what the yogic call mindfulness — and it's what happens to me in the kitchen."*

Beyond being a collection of recipes, this is a book about living. Ellen is like having an elfin, white, Jewish, vegan Oprah whispering in your ear that "it's going to be more than okay, honey — it's going to be *magical!*"

Another favorite I starred in the margin of my copy:

"Every time I start to write about faith,
I wind up writing about food."

A word to my fellow omnivores: you will find yourself *not* looking at this as a vegetarian cookbook that inherently contains restraints. Ellen would giggle and pinch you...metaphorically, at least! Her voice and wisdom roll off the pages without a bit of guilt-inducement or condescension. She is a seeker, not a proselytizer. She is here to awaken a more positive self in each of us. And I'm ready.

I'm also ready to have her gift me with the Ethiopian custom called *gursha* (see page xix). It is an act of friendship that translates as "hand-feeding." And I hope her Haitian Soupe Joumou (see page 12) is in the ancient spoon her gifted hand is holding when the *gursha* comes my way.

Come to think of it...it has already.

— Norman Van Aken,
coauthor (with Justin Van Aken) of *My Key West Kitchen*

Introduction

HUNGRY ALL *the* TIME

Eating — we do it every day; you'd think we'd have it down by now. And yet I hear from readers all the time who say they want a closer, healthier relationship with what they eat, with the planet, and with themselves. This should not be so hard. But it is.

I gave a talk recently, fashioned to be a sort of green's greatest hits. I wanted my audience to understand the consequences of what we eat, and why that might make them consider eating more produce and less meat. They might even go vegan. It happens. My talking points went something like this:

1. A meatless diet is cool, and not just because celebs are doing it; it's cool in terms of carbon output.
2. It's good for our health. The USDA's new dietary guidelines say so.
3. Even D. H. Lawrence got into it (at which point I threw in his line about figs being "glittering, rosy, moist, honied,"

to get the audience revved up about the connection between produce and pleasure).

People nodded. I had them. I ended big: change what you eat,
then change your life, then change the world. Applause. Then I
opened it up to questions.

A guy in the third row asked, "What do I eat for dinner?"

Excellent question. Because you can't change the world when
you can't even figure out what to eat at the end of a long day.

The French paradox enables the French to eat lavish, leisurely, artery-clogging meals while remaining svelte and chic,
with cholesterol levels that don't make their doctors scream and
hurl statins at them. The American paradox, by contrast, is just
depressing. We know more than we ever have before about what
our bodies and our planet need — yet we're in an obesity epi-
demic, and the earth isn't doing so great, either. March is National
Nutrition Month, but March 14 is National Potato Chip Day.
We're spending billions on diet books while consuming over a
million Twinkies a day. I myself do not participate in this Twinkie
fest, so don't look at me.

We watch food shows and follow celebrity chefs, but we don't
cook. Many of us don't even know how to shop for food, let alone
what to eat. One friend uses her oven as a shoe closet. Since she
doesn't cook, she eats as though on an endless campout — processed sausage, packaged cookies, chips, candy, and cinnamon
buns-o-rama, washed down with double mocha lattes, extra whip.
She's on a strict diet of nitrates, fat, and sugar, absent fruit and
vegetables. A whole grain never crosses her lips.

This is a girl who knows better. I'm thinking you know better, too. Knowing better is easy. Making changes armed with that

knowledge is what's hard, a bring-you-to-your-knees kind of hard. Sometimes it doesn't even seem possible. But it is.

My friend is wonderful, brilliant, beautiful, the best person I know. I'm just ninety-six pounds' worth of nervous. I worry about her. I worry about that guy, the one who doesn't know what to eat for dinner. I worry about you, too. Because you're probably as baffled as Mr. What's-for-Dinner and on the same diet my friend is on. Maybe you're not into cinnamon buns, but we're all caught up in today's frantic pace, fast food, big talk, empty calories, and empty promises — a diet of living that leaves us hungry and unfulfilled.

You deserve nourishment — nourishment from the food you eat, of course, but also from connection, balance, radiant good health, and the fun that seems to be happening at a party to which you were not invited. Hate that.

All the books and articles about weight loss and feeling better are great as far as they go. But to me, that's not far enough. Our relationship with food goes beyond a single meal or even a meal plan. Where food comes from, how it binds us to the planet and to each other, and how it makes us feel, matter more than what's on the plate. The things we hunger for — comfort, unconditional love, connection, meaning — aren't on the usual menu.

I think feeding that deeper hunger and serving the world start with what you serve for dinner. It means thinking beyond what's on your plate. It means seeing food as something that strokes the soul as it stokes the body, food as connection to and communion with the earth and each other. That's asking a lot of dinner. Get used to it. Asking a lot is what I do.

In elementary school, I was the annoying kid in class, arm raised, always asking why:

Why do people smoke/wage war/do drugs/have unpro-
tected sex if we know it's bad for us?

Why did we take America from the Indians when they
were here first?

Why is Jenny Slater in the bathroom crying?

I still ask a lot of questions, especially the big, cosmic kind.
I'm convinced our food holds the answers. I'm *Huffington Post's*
Meatless Monday blogger and a syndicated columnist, the Edgy
Veggie. I'm plant based by passion and profession; but don't get
weirded out by this detail, please. Think of me as the vegan who's
inviting everyone to the table.

I'm not a self-styled guru, a nutritional wonk, a New Ager,
an earth mother, a pedant, a product peddler, or a proselytizer.
I'm a fourth-generation Floridian who loves broccoli, and loves
being vegan but isn't hard-assed about it. I have sex with nonveg-
ans — at least one, my husband, Benjamin, an amazingly patient
man. Married to me, he would have to be. We have a mixed marriage. I am vegan to the max; he is an exuberant omnivore. We
work it out. Call it crazy love. We have no history of interesting
addictions, trauma, arrests, or experiences in rehab. We're not
devoutly anything, but we're well and living in Miami.

Miami is not exactly a bastion of the faithful, which explains
some of our collective quirks. It is many faiths and a lot of secular — and a little crazy-from-the-heat nuttiness. Miami sits at
the bottom tip of Florida, and Florida is at the bottom tip of the
United States. It has a history of attracting people who've tanked
out their other options and have run away as far as they can. Go
much farther south and you hit water.

Florida's best-known Catholic priest made tabloid headlines a
few years back by disporting himself on the beach with a woman.

The media had a feeding frenzy. Sinner! Hypocrite! Bad guy! The Catholic Church was not too happy, either. I was not one of his parishioners, but I thought, hey, given the recent filth uncovered in the church, a priest and an age-appropriate woman in love does not seem the worst thing in the world. Amid the media shouting, the priest reminded us there's a deeper, more complicated story, the one that comes of being human. That means we're all prone to messing up. "God's not all that interested in you falling down," he said. "God is interested in you getting up again."

This is a divine spirit I understand, someone I'd love to have over for dinner. I just can't wrap my brain around a divine spirit who's vengeful and pissed. Not that we don't try God's patience forty times before breakfast. Funny, every time I start to write about faith, I wind up writing about food.

Feeding the Hungry Ghost takes its title from the Tao concept of restless souls still hungry, still seeking, even beyond the grave. In ancient Buddhist scrolls, hungry ghosts are edgy, depicted as bug-eyed, big-bellied, and fierce. Wouldn't you be if you'd been staggering around for centuries without getting what you need? Hungry ghosts are assuaged by prayer and food. The same things do the trick for hungry mortals, too. We are hungry for so much more than food. But you know, like the guy at my talk, we'd all be glad to have something good to eat, too, and not have to struggle.

Even as we tweet endlessly about mindful eating, we have grown more disconnected from our food. Frankly, mindful eating sounds like a chore. But what if it felt like hanging out with a friend, one who feeds you terrific things, maybe even one who pops a bit of moist, velvety, and winningly dark chocolate cake in your mouth and then explains that hand-feeding is an Ethiopian custom of friendship and kinship known as *gursha*. That's what I want *Feeding the Hungry Ghost* to be.

To discuss food without discussing our relationship to it, be it ties to a recipe, to the culture, place, or time it comes from, or even to the pleasure of food itself, is to miss the bigger picture. Saffron, tarragon, cardamom, and cumin make food taste better. Culture, connection, and faith do the same thing for our lives. They make it delicious. They feed us.

I'm not here to enroll you in the Hungry Ghost Boot Camp. I won't attend a boot camp, let alone run one. I am more inclined to want to learn when not being shouted at or forced to wear unattractive footgear. And I am not into lies. You know, Change Your Life and Save the Planet in Five Steps and that whole genre. Because change takes a few steps more than five, and the hunger that needs feeding is something profound. So honor it. Honor yourself. I do. That's why I don't prescribe steps (or follow them). I prefer to be coaxed, gently nudged.

You have to eat every day, anyway, so you might as well fall in love with the right stuff. Why is our relationship with food important? For the same reason being alive is important. Because it is. Because you're here, so you might as well go for the whole delicious, authentic experience. Perhaps you subscribe to Thomas Hobbes's belief that life is nasty, brutish, and short. Honey, I've had days where I'd find it hard to disagree. But the thing is, it doesn't all suck. There's you, right? And you're not so bad.

And since you're here, alive and kicking, you might as well feel good. My wonderful friend is one of over a hundred million Americans who, despite their wonderfulness, have stratospheric cholesterol levels. Being wonderful does not make you exempt from the troubles of life. The trick is having the resources to handle them. It means nourishing every bit of yourself, soulfully and emotionally as well as nutritionally. I'll coax and gently nudge you along the path and cheer you on, every step of the way.

Can you do it? Hell, yeah. It's not only possible — it's energizing and delectable. We're not talking diet; we're talking about feeding our deepest hunger, for a more vital self, for more loving and meaningful connections, for a nourished and nourishing world, and yes, for fabulous food. That's what to eat for dinner. It's all interconnected. And it all adds up.

I've divided *Feeding the Hungry Ghost* into four chapters to help corral all this faith/food talk:

1. The Seed (for January, February, and March)
2. The Flowering (for April, May, and June)
3. The Harvest (for July, August, and September)
4. The Compost (for October, November, and December)

The earth has its rhythms, times of growth and bounty, of quiescence and regeneration. We call them seasons. Seasons are the way the world speaks to us. It even tells us what to eat, with trees providing juicy fruit to cool and hydrate us in summer, when it's hot; and dense, durable root vegetables grown from deep within the earth to sustain and nourish us in winter, when it's cold.

You have your own seasons, too. We all do — the darker days, when life reveals itself in all its sharp edges, and bright days of delicious joys. The calendar offers a way to start the conversation, but the main topic is you. And what to eat for dinner. We're all hungry. So let's begin.

a NOTE *on the* RECIPES

Life gives us many reasons to stress. Making dinner shouldn't add to them. I think of a recipe as a GPS — it's the directions to get you where you want to go, the end result being something that makes you smile and sigh as you eat and gives you the sense the world is looking out for you. At the very least, a recipe should enable you to create the fixings for a meal that tastes great and isn't a headache to make.

When a recipe here calls for a carrot or an onion, I mean any carrot or onion you can get your hands on without a struggle. If it's local, farmers'-market fresh, and organic, terrific. If it's slightly past its prime and you can't remember how it wound up in your kitchen in the first place, I'm delighted to give you a way to use it up. Unless otherwise indicated in a recipe, I'm not picky about the carrot's size, color, variety, or provenance. I leave that up to you. Likewise for the size of chopped bits. I'm attracted to crunch, texture. I like to see the components that go into my meal. Others prefer food finely chopped, diced, minced, or mirepoixed until their food achieves a sort of oneness. Go with what you like.

Say a particular recipe in this book really appeals to you. You look at the list of ingredients, and they're all among your pet delights. Except you're missing one item. So what are you going to do? It's the end of another workday, and you're already out of your elegant if constraining office wear and into your comfy wouldn't-be-caught-dead-going-out-in-public wear. Do not go food shopping on my account — go swapping. Feel free to substitute ingredients. Use what you have. Quinoa or another whole grain can pinch-hit for bulgur; scallions can stand in for an onion. It may not be as written, but it will still be fine. All will be well, you'll have prepared a meal you can cozy up to and enjoy, and you'll have no tears to dry.

Sometimes while you're following a recipe on the road to dinner, you find side paths, back roads that beckon and lead you to new places. Feel free to try a different vegetable, another herb. Take the road less traveled by, as Robert Frost put it. Go, explore. Strike out on your own. The recipe will work fine your way, my way, any way. Honor yourself and your own taste. Trust your gut.

I'm serious about cooking, about its adding pleasure, meaning, and connection to our lives. I am relaxed in my approach to it and hope you will be, too.

The recipes in this book aren't processed; they're primal. They embrace all cultures and are made from real food from the earth, food that goes back centuries. These dishes connect us with the past, with each other. And since many involve whole grains and beans, they're high in protein and fiber, and low in cash outlay — always a plus. Making and eating these dishes won't make you see God, but they may return you to the ability to see and hear your own not insignificant spirit. And that alone could change the world. Now go. Cook. Eat.

1 *the* SEED

Seeds are where it all begins. They promise the start of things. They're superconcentrated sources of energy. I look at everything growing in my backyard, from my newly sprouted purslane to the ten-foot firebush exploding with firecracker-red flowers, favorite of zebra longwing butterflies and humming-birds, to our thirty-foot live oak, which stretches its lanky, leafy limbs out to provide shelter and canopy. They all began as seeds — everyday magic.

Nature makes that kind of magic easy. You drop a seed in the dirt, cover it with soil, give it some water, leave the sun and the seed to make friends with each other, and honey, you're in business.

But then there's the fine print. Firebush needs direct sun and can handle shallow, sandy South Florida soil. It's a tough native. Purslane is supposed to be a weed and thus thrive like a weed, but mine's anemic, timid, probably suffering from sunstroke. Even weeds have their needs, and purslane prefers filtered sunlight. A seed only fulfills its superhero potential if it gets proper nurturing.

Then there are your more metaphoric seeds (and I do love a metaphor), the new beginnings life offers you — the joy of a new job, a new love, a new home, a new baby, a new year. Such new beginnings endow you with all the energy of a seed. You're awakening, feeling your way, tentatively reaching your roots into the soil. These kinds of seeds are times of hope; but they're always times of change, and change is tough.

Here's what's even tougher — you don't always get to choose a new beginning. Losing your job or breaking up with your partner wouldn't make anyone's list of top ten fave life events, but suddenly, there you are, in it up to your adenoids. That seed generates an energy of its own — like a tornado, it rips up your life and knocks you on your ass. It takes a herculean effort to roll out of bed in the morning. Where's the joy in that, ace?

And while it seems to be raining seeds around you, both the happy kind and the seeds you wouldn't even wish on your ex, think of yourself as a seed, too — a really gorgeous, spectacular, one-of-a-kind seed. But your gorgeousness can't come into full flowering unless you, too, get the nurturing you need.

For me, it means rooting myself in my community, being part of the initiatives that bring real food and real people together. Sometimes, I confess, I need to force myself to attend this meeting, that event. But I'm almost always better for it. The people I meet inspire me and energize me and take me in directions I didn't know I wanted to go. You're growing oyster mushrooms? Wow, how do you do that? How can *I* do that? You're teaching children to cook? Can I volunteer? I'm lucky to be nourished by my native soil.

You know best what kind of metaphoric soil you need, where you feel your happiest, truest self, where your own strength is coaxed forth, where you can set down strong roots and lift your face to the sun.

Or maybe you don't know. Maybe you've been so pelted with misery seeds, you barely know what you look like, let alone what you need. They say suffering is wonderfully character building. I say you've got plenty of character as it is. I say whatever's giving you grief should just get out of your way and get out of town. Until it does, though, you're stuck. You're going through hell, it's taking every ounce of your strength, and you can't quite see how you're ever going to return to that blissful, faraway place called normal.

Start by nurturing yourself. A basic way to give yourself the care you need is to pay attention to what you eat and to make healthier choices for all concerned — for you, for the planet.

Seeds are an easy place to begin. While vegetables still have their detractors (why? *why?*), anyone can chomp on a handful of seeds. If you're struggling, they'll support you nutritionally and offer a sprinkle of badly needed cheer. If you're happy, they'll only make you happier. They offer a crunch that bespeaks indulgence, but with it come the phytonutrients and fats our bodies hunger for, the kind that give us a nice inner glow, no microdermabrasion required.

Some seeds we snarf — sunflower seeds, pepitas (pumpkin seeds).

Some seeds we use to impart deep flavor in cooking — cumin, cardamom, mustard, coriander, fennel, to name a few of my favorites.

Some we eat without even realizing what they are. All your legumes, from teensy red lentils to massive gigantes are, botanically speaking, seeds.

And some we mean to get around to trying, because we hear

how tremendous they are for our health, yet we're daunted by them — flax, chia, and hemp come to mind.

Well, honey, your time has come. Whether you're flourishing or faltering, you need more of these teensy guys in your life. Flax rules when it comes to omega-3s, those excellent fatty acids. Chia seeds are right up there in the omega-3 department, but they also have a fantastic amount of fiber and antioxidants. Ancient Aztec warriors thrived on them, and they were pretty tough guys. Hemp seeds, tiniest of all, offer more protein per ounce than any animal protein.

Use them individually or mixed together in a seedy cocktail as a topping for casseroles and roasted vegetables. We love texture. Add them to grain dishes, both sweet and savory — oatmeal isn't oatmeal for me without a sprinkling of seeds. And chia and flax make excellent egg substitutes in baking. Mixing the seeds with a little water forms a bonding agent. Not only do you get the body-supporting benefit of the seeds; you get the nice cohesive quality of eggs without the cholesterol and without ruffling a single chicken feather.

SEED CAKE

I believe in backing up talk with something worth eating. So when I was thinking what kind of seedy recipe to use here, I thought of cake — seed cake, simple but soulful and long beloved in England, Ireland, and Scotland. Its origins date back as far as the Middle Ages, and back in the day, the seed in question tended to be caraway, making for a treat that walked the line between sweet and savory. Good as far as it goes, but trending toward heavy, and certainly heavy in vegan-unfriendly ingredients like butter, milk, and eggs.

Vegan baking, like life, is about balance and compromise.

Rather than weird you out with a bunch of arcane ingredients you'll have to shop for, I've swapped the traditional dairy and eggs for other items that are whole and plant based and fairly gettable. I've also swapped caraway seeds for anise. Like caraway, anise is excellent for digestion but has a gentler flavor. It's mildly licorice-y and is mellow in the mouth. It joins a symphony of other seeds for a moist cake of haunting fragrance and flavor.

Seed Cake

Serve as dessert or as an anytime restorative with coffee or tea.

Serves 8 or so

1 cup unsweetened soy or hemp milk

2 tablespoons ground flaxseeds (also known as flax meal)

2 tablespoons ground chia seeds

2 teaspoons anise seeds

1½ cups whole wheat flour

1 teaspoon baking soda

1 teaspoon aluminum-free baking powder

Zest and juice of 1 lemon

¾ cup evaporated cane sugar[*]

⅓ cup hemp, flax, or canola oil, plus more for the pan

½ cup unsweetened applesauce

⅓ cup raisins

---

[*] Less processed than white sugar, evaporated cane sugar looks similar to light brown sugar. It's sold in natural food stores and in many supermarkets. It's the go-to sugar in all *Feeding the Hungry Ghost* recipes.

Preheat the oven to 350°F. Lightly oil an 8-inch round cake pan or a 9-x-5-inch loaf pan.

In a small bowl, combine the soy milk, flaxseeds, chia seeds, and anise seeds. Stir gently to combine and let sit while you assemble the other ingredients.

In a large bowl, sift together the whole wheat flour, baking soda, and baking powder. Add the lemon zest.

In another large bowl, stir together the evaporated cane sugar, hemp oil, applesauce, and lemon juice. Add to the flour mixture, along with the soy milk mixture, which, thanks to the seeds, will have thickened madly. Stir together, then fold in the raisins.

Pour into the prepared baking pan. Bake for 45 minutes, or until the cake is golden and puffed, and a tester inserted in the center comes away crumb-free and clean. You can also give it a gentle poke with a finger; it should spring back when baked through.

Remove from the oven and let cool. Wrapped well and refrigerated, the cake keeps for several days.

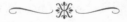

BIRTH *and* REBIRTH

If other species are aware of seasons of the year and hours of the day, they don't make a big deal about it. We humans, on the other hand, have arranged our lives around the calendar and the clock, all culminating at midnight, December 31, when all the days and nights of one year end and a new year begins. If that doesn't mark us as an interesting species, there's the fact that we observe this big do-over by drinking ourselves silly and kissing anything that moves.

When we wake up the next day, the world is hushed, quiet, curled in on itself, because after all, the planet hasn't partied like a fiend. It's feeling fine and doing what it always does — what any sane life form does — in the depth of winter: it rests, gathers strength, and waits for spring.

Not us, though. The New Year's Eve hangovers barely wear off before we're pacing our cages, eager to get back to the normal rhythm of our lives. And yet, we feel a heightened awareness and expectation. It's a new year! Everything feels new and fresh, and this is wonderful. Hope and the glimmering of possibility keep us light. Guilt and remorse weigh us down.

And yet guilt and remorse sell. We're attacked by ads shaming and shouting at us to lose all our holiday weight, join a gym, get six-pack abs. I've got nothing against a six-pack, but I hate all those "new you" things because I'm not so bad and you're lovely the way you are. And I hate cleansing diets, especially those sold in kits comprising little more than a bottle and a powdered, unpalatable mix of mystery ingredients.

A certain detox or dietary rethink is appropriate after the binging Bermuda Triangle of holidays (Thanksgiving, Christmas, New Year's Eve). However, I dislike being shouted at. The new year deserves to be entered gradually and gently, rather than dived into headlong, because the shock alone could kill you. Going from a month of party foods to a diet solely composed of lemon and water may help you pee off a few pounds, but it's nothing you can stick to, especially when it's bitter and gray outside. It exacts a toll on your body and soul. It makes you cranky and weak.

Winter tends to make me cranky, anyway. Yes, even in Miami. On a bad day, when the wind bites through my pathetic idea of a warm jacket, the one that makes me look like a homeless person with no fashion sense, when I'm frazzled by deadlines and deadbeats, the new year reveals itself to be pretty much like last year, with all the baggage, all the stress, but without December's sparklies and parties, plus a massive holiday credit card bill to pay off. It's fine for the tourists to go around in their wifebeaters and shorts, flip-flops and sunburns; but it is winter in my soul, and it's hard to feel the benevolent force in, well, just about anything.

This is a good time to go back to bed. Until April. A normal person would sleep. I bury myself in blankets, dutifully close my eyes. They pop open. I'm so rigid with tension, I all but levitate. My brain will not shut up. "So, Ellen," it says in that snarky tone it gets when I'm vulnerable. "What happened to your big plans for this shiny new year? You know, achieving world peace, solving global food scarcity. Where are you with those? From here, it looks like you're just lying there. Wasting time."

I have made absurd, unattainable New Year's resolutions. And they only wind up frustrating me and making me feel like a loser. So for quite a few years now, I've resolved to embrace chaos. Because it's coming at us whether we like it or not. I'm still not great at it but have grown more comfortable with the concept; there are things in the world beyond my personal control — oil spills, war, hunger, illness, stuff like that. I hate that I can't fix these things, but I am learning to be — oh, who am I kidding? I'll always worry. I don't like to worry, but I'm good at it. However, because I'm learning to embrace chaos, I'm okay with my own worry. I can even let some of it go. A little. Then I worry some more.

I envy people who take comfort in faith — the defined, institutional kind — that God will provide, or if something really wretched happens, it's okay because it's God's will, or — inshallah — that it will happen as Allah wishes. These are especially the times I'd like to ask God, Allah, or whoever's in charge, just what the hell he's after.

I'm not entirely sure I believe in God. I understand he/she

believes in me, which I find most cheering. I think if there is a God, it's bighearted despite our quirks and craziness, able to focus on the big picture, see what we're doing and basically shrug and say, "Oy, what can you do?" I was raised Jewish, but Reform. Really Reform. My husband, Benjamin, thinks my family's so Reform, we deserve another category — Mellow. Benjamin was raised Lutheran, and in his childhood did refined things I associate with WASP-dom. He attended cotillion. His family ate Jell-O salads. They belonged to a yacht club.

But in both his case and mine, the formal religion part just didn't take. What resonates with Benjamin about Judaism is latkes. At every Jewish holiday, he asks, "Is this the potato pancake one?" What resonates with me is the more secular part of Judaism, the concept of *tikkun olam*, healing the world, the social responsibility part.

Am I Jewish? According to liturgy, yes, but among the list of modifiers I'd choose, *vegan* and *female* would come well before it. Also *nervous*.

In each new year, I try, again, to come to terms with human frailty, mine, yours, big, small. When I come splat against yet another of my human limitations, I have an ungodly response. I get pissed.

Good karma takes way too long for me, but the karma of being pissed bites me right back in the ass every time. So I begin again. I need definite — and positive — intention. I can't just lie in bed and hope war will end. I need to take action.

For a long time, I thought the only way I could serve humanity was by running off and joining Doctors without Borders. Just how I, with no formal medical training, was going to help them was a little hazy.

So I started doing small, specific things that didn't require a visa or medical degree. I joined a massive volunteer effort to help kids plant an organic garden in their public school. We dug up the patchy sod — hard, hot, hand-blistering work. We planted the seeds. We grew fat, red tomatoes, glossy eggplant, and a tangle of greens including callaloo, a green gift from the Caribbean. I showed kids how to cook it. I watched them eat it — a vegetable!

The kids liked it, not because it was good for them, but because they made it happen, from planting the seed to harvesting it and braising it with chili and garlic. It's that sense of ownership, of hey, I've got a personal stake in this, that makes food taste good, that gives it value. It's all about connecting with how our food is grown and sourced, with the planet, and with that great big, mystical thing beyond it. The schoolkids discovered fresh produce; I discovered my own community and that I'm better at working and playing with kids than I'd led myself to believe.

Hanging out at the farmers' markets, belonging to our local community's shared agriculture program, working with some amazing chefs and organizations and initiatives that bring what our farmers grow to the people who need to eat it — this is my idea of a good time. I can't promise it brings me to salvation. But it helps bring me back to myself, plus I get to write about it and turn readers on to a good thing or two.

That's how I met my friend Marcel, genius of soup, specifically soupe joumou, the beloved soup with which Haitians start the new year. It's not enough for Marcel to make it; he has to feed everyone he knows. So he makes a vat of it on a hot plate in his studio and serves it up all day. Even in dark times.

The 2010 earthquake devastated his homeland. He lost his auntie, uncle, and cousins, all with a shake of the earth. This is when the fetal position comes in handy. Instead, Marcel wanted to make soup. He *needed* to make soup. When I arrived, his place was flooded with afternoon light and was so jammed, I couldn't see the host for all the guests clustered around him, cradling soup bowls, talking, eating, laughing.

Finally, I found Marcel in his makeshift kitchen, holding court and presiding over the soup pot.

I gave him a kiss and picked up a bowl.

"It has meat," he warned, remembering I'm a meat-free kind of girl.

"I'll eat around it."

We looked at each other. He beamed and ladled it, rich and golden, like liquid sunshine, from a battered aluminum pot.

Soupe joumou is the triumph of spirit over tyranny, heart over privation, and a damn fine way to warm body and soul. This is a soup tapping into the collective unconscious of a people, evoking stronger feelings than Proust's madeleine. I wasn't going to let some bits of beef get in the way of that.

We all love to ring in the new year with its promise of new beginnings, but in Haiti, it's especially cause for joy. New Year's Day is Independence Day, the celebration of that New Year's Day in 1804 when Haitians ended over a century of bloody rule by the French and were no longer colonial slaves, but a free people in their own country.

Haitians celebrated by eating what had been forbidden them — meat, cabbage, and squash, the latter two grown on their own island. Haitian slaves had grown and cooked these foods for their French masters, while they themselves had survived solely on rations of salt cod and lemonade.

Soupe joumou sustains and is sustainable. It's made from what is local and available. The Haitians adapted the soup from their French masters, heating it up with habaneros and ginger and making it their own. Some eat it on New Year's Day for good luck. Others, like Marcel, eat and serve it knowing its history. It is his connection to place and to people, his source of sanity and serenity.

As with all things Haitian, there is some myth involved. The soup is said to honor Papa Loko, the vodou god of the ancient African spirit. Yellow is his favorite color, the one that summons him. Soupe joumou summons everyone. It's belly filling and soul lifting all at once. It epitomizes for me the people of Haiti, who take what little they have, make it delicious, and offer it to you with all their heart.

It isn't that life hasn't lobbed a lot of crap Marcel's way or that he's weatherproofed against it. No one is. It's how we bear up that matters. And Marcel, on the anniversary of losing home and family, somehow managed with grace and made soup. That's enough of a superpower for me.

Haitian Soupe Joumou

I have swapped traditional winter squash for sturdier sweet potato and have taken the meat out of Marcel's soupe joumou. I have not, I hope, taken the heart. This Haitian dish is filling and satisfying. You need only add some nice crusty bread like No-Knead Whole Wheat Oatmeal Bread (page 182) or even Flatbread from a Starter (page 214) and you'll have a meal to make you happy.

Serves 4

1 tablespoon coconut oil
1 onion, chopped

¼ cup minced fresh garlic (yeah, ¼ cup — got a problem?)
¼ cup minced fresh ginger
1 jalapeño chili (or ¼ habanero chili), minced
1½ teaspoons ground allspice
1 sweet potato, chopped
2 carrots, chopped
1 bunch collard greens or callaloo, chopped into bite-size
     pieces
4 cups Stone Soup (see page 84) or other vegetable broth
1 teaspoon fresh thyme leaves
1 bay leaf
1 lime, halved
Sea salt and freshly ground pepper

Heat the coconut oil in a soup pot over medium-high heat. Add
the onion, garlic, ginger, and jalapeño. Sauté, stirring occasionally,
until the vegetables soften, about 8 minutes. Add the allspice, sweet
potato, and carrots. Add the collards, a handful at a time, and cook
until they just wilt, about 3 minutes. Add the broth and raise the
heat to high. When the broth comes to a boil, add the thyme leaves
and bay leaf. Reduce the heat to low, cover, and simmer for 30 minutes, or until the vegetables are tender. Squeeze the juice from the
lime over the top and season with sea salt and pepper.

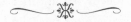

FEEDING FAITH

I think you can find faith in a temple or a mosque or a church,
but you can also find it in a garden or a school or studio, or in
a kitchen, like Marcel. That's where I find faith, too. Prayer is

attentiveness — what the yogic call mindfulness — and it's what happens to me in the kitchen.

Cooking is its own meditation. If you can sit on your ass, breathe deeply, and find balance and serenity, honey, I salute you. Me, I've got to move, and cooking is something I can do to keep my brain from spinning like a centrifuge. It helps me deal with the day-to-day crazies and still keep my eye on the prize, whatever the prize is. The converse applies, too. When work or life conspires to keep me out of the kitchen for a while, I get a little wiggy.

When I'm cooking, I know I can't cure cancer, can't impose my will on an unruly coworker or politician, can't make a deadline go away. Even on a bad day, though, I can make a big batch of something that pleases, comforts, and nourishes the people I love or that somehow connects me to them. Like when I make soupe joumou.

Everything must be done in a certain order. First, I chop the vegetables. Then I sauté them. I stir and watch as the garlic, onions, and ginger are gilded with oil and grow tender. I breathe in a smell both sweet and pungent. Focusing on each step and the physical action required brings me back to my core, to that teensy little place where I am sane and whence flows my belief that the universe is still a good place to be. And since you're here, stick around; I've got a great pot of soup in the works, too.

I have a religious fervor for another winter dish. It's nothing posh — just rice, black-eyed peas, and collards — but it's as satisfying as anything I've ever eaten. It whispers, "There, there, honey. Dinner's ready," while offering antioxidants, calcium, protein, and, thanks to the power of collard greens, outrageous amounts of vitamins K, A, and C. This New Year's Day tradition is cheapish to make and rich in fiber and folklore.

Just why it's called hopping john is sketchy. I've heard the dish got its name from a child dancing around the stove, eager for supper. I've also heard the recipe came from a man named John with a limp. They both sound like stories concocted after too much alcohol.

Most food historians believe the dish itself originated with the slaves who brought black-eyed peas and rice from west Africa. What started as a slave dish was livened with a little pepper and pork, and made its way into plantation kitchens.

Some say black-eyed peas look like coins and collards or other greens represent paper money; therefore, you'll make as much money as the hopping john you eat. Black-eyed peas also fit an old superstition that if a dark-eyed man is your first visitor on New Year's Day, love and luck will be yours.

Good luck, great fortune, and hot romance — I believe in all three. I don't quite believe a plate of rice and beans will make that happen. But just in case it will, I have a pot of hopping john ready every New Year's Day.

It fills us up yet opens up our hearts just the wee-est bit so we can let go of the hurt, the anxiety, the tightness, the meanness, all the dark, heavy things that were so last year.

Make it New Year's Eve or even the day before. The flavor improves over time, and hopping john reheats like a dream. And there's a bonus — the sturdy rice-and-beans dish sops up any hangover.

Dishes like hopping john and soupe joumou sustain the body because they're made with ingredients that are humble but whole, nutritious, and recognizable. They sustain the soul because they have a rich cultural and culinary history. They connect us to our past and to each other. This is the real meaning of soul food. It's food that's meant to be shared, that lets you know you're not alone in the universe. And if that's not religion, I don't know what is.

Hopping John

Hopping john makes a comforting one-pot meal, and with its lure, lore, and luck, stands alone. However, a green salad makes a nice, fresh counterpoint.

Traditionally, hopping john is made with pork. This version is pigless. Like it spicy? Me, too. Enjoy with a splash of your favorite hot sauce.

Serves 6

1 cup dried black-eyed peas
3 cups water
6 cloves garlic
1 dried red pepper, crumbled, or a pinch of red pepper
    flakes
1 bay leaf
1 cup brown rice
2 cups Stone Soup (see page 84) or other vegetable broth
1 tablespoon olive oil
1 large onion, chopped
1 jalapeño chili, minced
3 stalks celery, chopped
1 bunch collard greens, chopped into bite-size pieces
1 lemon, halved
Sea salt and freshly ground pepper

Black-eyed peas, like most dried beans, benefit by overnight soaking. It makes them tender to eat and easy to digest. Start with my master plan for cooking dried beans. Pour beans into a bowl, cover with cold water and just leave them alone until the next day. Drain the beans and rinse.

In a large pot, bring the 3 cups water to a boil over high heat. Add the black-eyed peas, 2 cloves of the garlic, the dried red pepper, and the bay leaf. Skim off and discard any peas that float. They're duds. Reduce the heat to low and simmer, uncovered. The peas can be left alone. Don't stir them. Cooking time varies for dried beans. Let them cook until tender, not mushy. In the case of black-eyed peas, it'll take about 1½ hours.

Add the brown rice and the vegetable broth. Cover and simmer for 20 minutes more. Don't lift the lid. Turn off the heat, leave the pot on the stove top, and let the hopping john sit while you prepare the collard greens.

Mince the remaining 4 garlic cloves. Heat the olive oil in a large skillet over medium-high heat. Add the onion, jalapeño, celery, and minced garlic. Sauté, stirring occasionally, until the vegetables soften, about 5 minutes.

Reduce the heat to medium. Add the collards, a handful at a time, and cook until they just wilt, stirring occasionally, about 10 minutes.

Fluff the rice and black-eyed peas and fold in the collards mixture. Squeeze the juice from the lemon halves over the top, season with salt and pepper, and stir to combine.

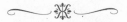

GENTLE NUDGE *the* FIRST: BUSINESS PLAN

You're a busy person. I can save you time: act and eat mindfully.

Don't close the book yet. Look, it needs a better name. Call it "Oprah" for all I care, *mindfulness* is really just a word for adding it up, for implementing a workable business plan. What do you want for yourself? What do you want for the planet? Now act accordingly.

For starters, think about what you're going to eat next. Make a conscious decision only to eat food you recognize.

No, for real.

This thing you're going to eat — what goes into making it? An apple is made from an apple seed, the soil where it's planted, sun, water, and the time it takes to grow. A brand-name fast-food apple fritter is made from refined white flour, high-fructose corn syrup, hydrogenated oil, and a whole lot of other things, including propylene glycol, which is used in antifreeze. It is only 2 percent apple.

Honey, eat the apple. Propylene glycol is just one of some seven thousand food additives, and the average American eats a dozen pounds of them a year. Additives are substances not naturally in what you're eating. They're put there by manufacturers who want to bling up their food so it looks prettier, tastes better, lasts longer.

Reading the label on packaging tells you something, but unless you spend your days in a lab, you probably bleep over the long chemical names and hope for the best. Hope's good. Knowledge doesn't hurt, either. Chances are, there's more in your Happy Meal than you realize.

Yes, it's a free world, a free country, and you can eat additives if you want to. But you're not here to do yourself harm. If you don't recognize the ingredient, don't put it in your body. Go for pure ingredients.

You can reduce your carbon footprint, reduce your waistline, boost your eco-awareness, boost your metabolism, feel a vital connection to all living things, get that natural-glow thing going, and save money all in one go. Wanna talk multitasking at its easiest?

Mindfulness is a process, a practice, a gradual awakening.

Be patient with yourself; you don't have to get it all down today. Relax. It's all part of the journey.

a CHILD'S GARDEN

The seeds of food and faith took root in me early, creating a rogue hybrid. I wasn't a voracious eater as a kid, but I was a voracious reader. I read books and stories and poems, but also street signs, cereal boxes, magazines, billboards, and ketchup labels. And cookbooks, which I read as though they were storybooks. Each recipe told a tale — the ingredients were the characters, the preparation was the plot, and every one was a total, page-turning thrill. Take cheese soufflé — could beating egg whites really transform the slimy, transparent stuff at the bottom of the bowl into something huge, white, and fluffy? And how could the egg whites lift and rescue the cheese sauce for the soufflé? Would they all live happily ever after? No way! It would all go wrong! The mysteries of the kitchen had to be plumbed. Also on my to-do list: the mysteries of life.

If I was hungry for anything, it was to discover everything about it *now*. There was so much to know, but at six, I could already tell I wasn't getting the real story. At school, at home, on TV, grown-ups were giving me the abridged, sanitized, G-rated version of life. I could tell by their wide, toothy smiles. I didn't buy their version of things for a red-hot minute.

Then my parents announced they were sending me to Sunday school. This presented definite downsides. It shot a hole in a perfectly good weekend. I had to wear dresses that mothers called "darling," which meant they itched and had fussy collars and I couldn't run around in them.

On the other hand, I sensed you could get to the bottom of

things at Sunday school. The temple sanctuary, with its high, vaulted ceiling and stained-glass windows, was cool, silent, and still. It was what wisdom felt like.

But we were kids, little ones, given to tantrums, noise, and mess. We were not allowed in the sanctuary. Instead, the teachers herded us into classrooms with buzzing fluorescent lights. They talked about holidays, made us sing songs, and gave out construction paper, glue, and crayons for crafts. At first, I bided my time. Maybe we had to pass some kind of test before they'd let us in on things. I was determined to prove myself worthy.

By the third year, though, it was clear — we'd been duped.

Well, if the Sunday school teachers weren't going to share the secrets of life, I was going to find out on my own. So one Sunday, as we went single file to art class, I stood at the back of the line. Instead of turning right, toward more paper, more crayons, more adult deception, I turned left. Over the pounding of my heart, I walked out of the classroom building, out of the temple, and into the whole world.

The whole wide world did not give up its mysteries easily. I passed a car dealership, an office building, and the field of patchy grass and crumbling masonry that is Miami's oldest cemetery. I was all alone, and my bravery had its limits. I ran past the cemetery, turned the corner, kept running — and found the S&S Diner.

The whole wide world is very big. The S&S is cozy. It has red awnings, big plate-glass windows, and no tables. It's all horseshoe counter, with red stools, the kind I loved to spin on, but there was no spinning going on inside; there were no kids. A couple sat together, laughing, their hands cradling mugs. Otherwise, people sat by themselves, plates and glasses and newspapers scattered around them, making a mess, resting their elbows on the counter, doing all the things I wasn't supposed to do. This was the most grown-up place in the world. And I was in it.

I squeezed the coins in my pocket, calculating if I had enough money for chocolate milk, when the waitress spotted me. "Well, hey there."

The diners looked over, then back at their plates. Except for one man. He kept staring at me. The rabbi.

Not the Nice Rabbi, the happy, young one the whole congregation loved, but the Real Rabbi, tall, gray haired, old, with thick-lensed glasses and no smile whatsoever.

He said, "Come here."

I have never been so busted in my life as I was at that moment. But it had never occurred to me before — rabbis ate. His breakfast didn't seem religious; it seemed normal grown-up — scrambled eggs, black coffee, toast.

"Why aren't you in class?" His breath smelled eggy.

I studied the plastic rack of little individual jellies and longed to arrange them by color and flavor preference.

"Dunno," I whispered.

"You...don't...know?"

He didn't have to threaten or torment me. I was not used to misbehaving, not good at it. I caved.

"I get bored."

The rabbi blinked. His glasses made his eyes look extra big. "Tell me," he said.

So I explained the songs and the crafts were not quite what I was after. I wanted to know why people have to die, where they go when they're dead, why bad things happen, and whether dogs could be Jewish.

He took a breath. So did I. The rabbi was a wise man; that was the whole deal. Would he level with me?

"Do you have a dog?" he asked. I nodded.

He broke a triangle of toast in half, spread a blob of purple jelly on it, and handed it to me. He hadn't cut off the crust. I took a bite anyway, away from the crust. Having been sitting there a while, the toast had gone cold, and the crunch was gone.

He said I was asking questions rabbis had been asking for ages. Even they didn't have all the answers. Well, what was the point of being a grown-up, of being a rabbi, if you didn't get to know everything? I think he said something about life being a process or a journey. He might as well have handed me a box of crayons.

"Tell me about your dog," he said. He asked about my family. He asked about me. He paid and we walked back to the temple, him looming above me.

Instead of dumping me back in class, he led me to the temple's library. It was empty inside and dark, but he flicked a switch and it glowed with light. There were just the two of us and the room of books, great big grown-up books, all lining the shelves and yearning to be read.

"You like to read. You're looking for answers. What if on days you don't want to go to class, instead of running away, you come here?" Then he said. "It can be our secret. Do we have a deal?"

I nodded. A secret was good. But knowing things was better. I would have to read a lot to learn everything. But I already knew more than the rabbi. He put grape jelly on his toast. Anyone knows raspberry's better.

With grown-ups and religion suddenly on my iffy list, I turned to poetry.

Poetry — okay, children's rhymes — shaped my thinking

about food far more than any diet phenom, veggie fest, or food show. I somewhere came across Walter de la Mare's poem "Miss T.," which begins, "It's a very odd thing — / As odd as can be — / That whatever Miss T. eats / Turns into Miss T."

This was mind altering for me, like kiddie LSD. Of course food literally goes into you when you eat it, but I realized it *becomes* you, too. Whatever you eat gets integrated into your very essence. You literally *are* a warming bowl of oatmeal or a handful of neon-orange cheese curls, a fresh strawberry, or a slab of meat loaf.

The message of "Miss T.," delivered for the under-eight set, is very much like the famed aphorism of eighteenth-century French gastronome Jean Anthelme Brillat-Savarin — "Tell me what you eat, and I shall tell you what you are." I can't draw a straight line between my very vegan self now and the little girl revved by words and rhymes, but that poem, with its clever cadence and fanciful images, made me think about what I ate. So did Florence Page Jaques's poem "There Once Was a Puffin."

The poem's bird hero, with its sad clown face, lived all alone on an island, without "anybody to play with at all." I would have been happy to play with the puffin. Instead, I worried. Where was the rest of his flock? Had they moved on? Why would they do that? And *how* did they do that? Didn't they realize puffins can't fly?

There were more worries ahead, in the following stanzas. The puffin hung out and ate fish, but he was lonely. Until the fish came and made him an offer — "You can have us for playmates, / Instead of for tea!" Then everything got better, and they all became friends. Now "the Puffin eats pancakes, / Like you and like me."

Happy ending, on to the next poem. But like "Miss T.,"

"There Once Was a Puffin" stayed with me. Woven into the lilting rhyme scheme was a seed, a lesson about compassionate eating. It's best not to eat your friends. Especially when you can have pancakes instead.

Whole Grain Pancakes

Timing is everything. While many recipes in this book will encourage you to take your time, pancakes will wait for no one. Make the batter just before cooking and heat the griddle or skillet as hot as you can. You will be rewarded with fluffy cakes that aren't half bad — or half bad for you.

Serve with maple syrup, fresh fruit, powdered sugar, or whatever you like. You can even serve these topped with sautéed vegetables, in which case it'll be a more substantial and brunchy affair. A puffin would approve.

Makes about one dozen 3-inch pancakes

1 tablespoon vegan margarine, such as Earth Balance, plus
    more for cooking the pancakes
1 cup unbleached all-purpose flour
¼ cup whole wheat flour
¼ cup old-fashioned oats (also known as rolled oats)
1½ teaspoons aluminum-free baking powder
1 teaspoon ground flaxseeds (also known as flax meal)
1¾ cups plain or vanilla soy milk

Melt the 1 tablespoon vegan margarine in a large skillet; set aside. Meanwhile, combine the all-purpose flour, whole wheat flour, oats, baking powder, and flaxseeds in a large bowl. Add the soy milk and the melted vegan margarine to the dry ingredients and stir until just combined — do not maul or manhandle the batter.

Melt additional vegan margarine in the skillet over high heat. Pour or ladle about ¼ cup of the pancake batter onto the griddle to form a 3-inch pancake. Add as many more pancakes to the pan as you can fit, allowing plenty of room between them.

Cook until the edges brown and a few bubbles form, about 4 minutes. Using a flexible spatula, flip the pancakes and cook until golden brown and fluffy, about 4 to 5 minutes.

Serve at once.

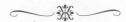

Enjoy. Me, I am not a true eater of pancakes. I am not a true eater of breakfast (perhaps we can blame the rabbi incident). Or rather, I don't eat breakfast in the morning. I like it much later in the day. A bowl of oats with cinnamon, flaxseed, and walnuts, or a sexy, slickery mango, or a just-baked muffin and a cup of coffee or tea. What could be bad? This is a quirk or predilection — a much nicer word — I picked up from my grandmother Marcella.

My mother dutifully, lovingly cooked most of my meals when I was growing up, but it was Marcella who taught me more about eating. And adventure. She was my paternal grandmother, a Kanner not by blood but by marriage, who, thank God, injected the Kanner line with a much-needed dose of liveliness and mischief. I have a good many Kanner traits. I give bad phone. I have a telegram-like terseness, a tendency toward thinness, good teeth, good feet, and an amazing capacity to feel cold even in Miami. But from my grandmother, I get a love of the exotic and, alas, an inability to filter. Like her, I tend to blurt inappropriate things.

Marcella could not cook. When I was little, her scrambled

eggs — overdone, brown, rubbery — made me cry. She was renowned for her vile coffee, watery yet corrosive. She was not your traditional grandmotherly type with a soft and available lap. Back in the 1920s, Marcella had road-tripped from Florida to California with her soon-to-be sister-in-law, my great-aunt Rose, the fussiest woman on earth. How they managed is anyone's guess. There was no getting to the bottom of it when I'd ask them, and there's no one alive to tell the tale now.

Marcella married and became a mother and then grandmother, but she never quite settled down. She smoked and drank and played cards with the girls — even when she and "the girls" were well into their seventies. The most grandmotherish thing Marcella did was knit, but she was keener on golf and swimming, and had a swimmer's broad shoulders and a thrill seeker's nature. For Marcella, the spirit of adventure came naturally; it was part of who she was. In me, it needed cultivating. I was a shy, bookish little girl of seven, and my idea of adventure was getting lost in stories. I'd been in an acute *Tales of a Thousand and One Nights* phase when I wound up in Marcella's tow one afternoon while she ran errands. We went to the yarn store, where bosomy women pinched my cheeks (why do they *do* that?), to the dry cleaner, with its chemical smells and the racks of clothes spinning from the ceiling, and finally to a place I'd never seen before — a Middle Eastern grocery.

It must have been the only one in Miami at the time. It was small, dim, with narrow aisles lined with shelves stacked high with bags and bottles and jars of things totally mysterious to me. And yet somehow not mysterious. I knew this place. I knew it from *Tales of a Thousand and One Nights*.

My heart pounded as I peered about for Scheherazade in gauzy robes and bangles. But the only other person in the store was the slightly terrifying owner, who regarded us from beneath a ledge of bushy black eyebrows. I wanted to rub every jar in the store, to find one that conjured a djinn, or at least plunge my hands into the bins of lentils and bulgur, sweeping them up and letting them fall, like playing in sand without the beach. But the owner scowled, and I didn't dare. Disapproval came off him as sharp as the scent of sumac and feta, which mingled with the other smells in the store — tangy, cured grape leaves, heady saffron, sweet cardamom.

I slipped my hand into my grandmother's. Clearly, we had left the sanctity and security of the known world. It didn't bother my grandmother any. From one of the bins, she measured out a scoop of the dried apricots she loved to snack on, curled and furrowed like little ears, but sweet and tart and chewy. She asked the owner for some feta, which he kept in a refrigerated case, an immense white cake bobbing in its own briny bath. She also asked for a wedge of something that sat next to it, a mound of something tan. He sliced it and was about to wrap it up in butcher paper, when she reached over and broke off a piece right there in the shop.

I braced for the man to produce a scimitar and hack us into bits.

My grandmother, oblivious, gave me a nugget. "It's halvah."

So this was to be my last meal. I ate it. It was both like and unlike anything I'd ever tasted. It was sweet, it was peanut buttery, it was just a little bit gritty, then whoom, it dissolved in my mouth and was gone. I instantly wanted more.

"Halvah," I said. And the name was sweet in my mouth as well, a magical incantation. The owner ceased glowering and beamed.

You could say halvah was my gateway drug. From then on, I was always game to try new foods, and Marcella was happy to be my guide. Baba ghanoush, one of her favorites, was an easy sell. It's garlicky, yes, and unlovely but has a name like one of Scheherazade's heroes. Guacamole, which Marcella insisted on calling "guamacole," was a staple during summer when her avocado tree bore abundantly. I came to like it after she let me make it with her. I squished the avocado between my fingers; she rubbed bits of it on her face — free moisturizer.

Then came my grandmother's beloved limburger. My grandfather banned it from the house. Or tried to. Marcella kept it tightly sealed in a jar at the back of the fridge and only let it out — like a bad djinn — when he was away. She'd phone out of the blue and say, "Your grandfather's out. Let's have lunch." This meant limburger and onion sandwiches on pumpernickel, a combination that makes my eyes water just thinking of it.

Or maybe my eyes water because Marcella died years ago and we are no longer each other's gastronomic partner in crime. I miss the way her eyes lit up with pleasure when I introduced her to something new, like Indian lemon pickle — too much salt, too much chili, too much oil, can I have some more, please? I wish she were still alive so she could try pomegranate molasses, puckery and intense, but with a sweet finish. Or natto — pungent fermented soybeans — a Japanese dish that gives limburger a run for its money. I wish I could make her kimchi and harissa, their flavors fierce, fiery, tangy, offering bright flashes from other lands.

My grandmother traveled the country; I travel the globe. She was a passionate eater. I'm a passionate eater and cook. I feel her presence at Ecuadoran cevicherías, in Moroccan souks, and in my kitchen when I make harissa and halvah. I can imagine her peering into bowls and dipping her finger in to taste.

What I loved about *Tales of a Thousand and One Nights* was that it did not end. Stories opened up into other stories. Food is the same way. One culinary adventure leads into the next, and the djinn can be anywhere — in a Moroccan tagine, a Turkish *guvec*, their names almost as magical as *halvah*, or just as easily in a great pot of coffee you share with someone you love.

Turkish Millet and Greens for Marcella

Offering whole grains, fabulous greens, and haunting flavors, this dish is a one-pot wonder. However, if you feel it would be lonely by itself, it pairs very nicely with fennel. A side dish of roasted fennel drizzled with balsamic vinegar has a nice chewiness. For a crisp contrast, shred raw fennel or enjoy the millet with the Pink Grapefruit and Fennel Salad (page 39).

Serves 6 to 8

¾ cup walnuts

2½ cups Stone Soup (see page 84) or other vegetable broth
     or water

1 cup millet

2 tablespoons olive oil

1 large onion, chopped

4 cloves garlic, thinly sliced

1 to 2 teaspoons red pepper flakes, or 1 or 2 dried red
     peppers, crumbled

1 bunch greens (collards, kale, chard — whatever's green
     and fresh), chopped into bite-size pieces

⅓ cup finely chopped fresh dill

One 15-ounce can diced tomatoes

2 tablespoons tomato paste

½ cup pomegranate molasses*
1 teaspoon ground coriander
Sea salt and freshly ground pepper
1 bunch fresh cilantro, chopped

Preheat the oven to 350°F. Coarsely chop the walnuts and pour into a shallow baking pan. Bake until they're golden brown and have a wonderful buttery smell, about 10 minutes. Set aside to cool.

In a large saucepan, bring the vegetable broth to a boil over high heat. Add the millet. Cover, reduce the heat to low, and simmer until all the liquid is absorbed, about 20 minutes.

Fluff the cooked millet with a fork and set aside to cool. (The cooked millet can be stored in an airtight container in the refrigerator for a day or two; bring to room temperature before proceeding with the recipe.)

In a large pot, heat the oil over medium-high heat. Add the onion, garlic, and red pepper flakes. Cook, stirring occasionally, until the vegetables are fragrant and softened, about 8 minutes.

Add the greens, a handful at a time, and the dill, and cook until the greens just wilt, stirring occasionally, 3 to 5 minutes. Add the walnuts, cooked millet, and tomatoes, stirring gently to keep the millet clump-free. Stir in the tomato paste and pomegranate molasses. Add the coriander, stir to combine, and season with salt and pepper. (The millet and greens can be stored in an airtight container in the refrigerator for a day or two; reheat just before serving.)

Stir in the cilantro just before serving.

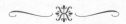

---

* Pomegranate molasses is available at Middle Eastern markets and many gourmet stores.

GENTLE NUDGE *the* SECOND: DISCOVER *the* POWER *of* LITERATURE — YOUR OWN

I kept a diary in my teens, chronicling my angst and misadventures and brain-bending crushes. It was, of course, puerile, self-absorbed, all of it. But you know what Oscar Wilde said — "I never travel without my diary. One should always have something sensational to read in the train."

It's time you kept a diary, too — a food diary, where you record everything that goes in your mouth. What could be more sensational than you?

The hardest part of sticking to a food regimen — or any regimen — is the human factor. We lie to ourselves. All the time. A nicer way to say this is we fudge — oh, dangerous, delicious word — on the truth. We cheat. We start out great guns, but then we cave. We get tired, bored, cranky, tempted.

I can't keep you honest. That ain't in my pay grade. A food journal will do the work for you. Do it for real for one month, and you'll have something more thrilling than a Kardashian tell-all, and more authentic besides. It'll reveal your own eating behavior.

According to the dog whisperer who trains both our wayward puppy and me, there's always a behavior pattern. We all have blind spots, things we rationalize. The trick is to keep notes so you can recognize yours. So watch and learn.

Don't judge yourself, don't forbid yourself anything, especially food you love and associate with comfort (because why else would you eat it?). But when you start seeing how much you eat and when — what the behaviorists call triggers — you may come to that aha moment and feel ready to make some tweaks. That's how I got myself off my soda jones.

Uh, yeah. Full and shaming disclosure — I used to drink

soda, your worst dietary offender. And I used to drink a lot of it — close to two liters a day. I justified drinking it the way we all justify bad habits: could be worse, I could be an ax murderess, so what's so bad about a can of soda?

Well, for one thing, that's where a lot of calories and sugar are. According to a University of North Carolina study, we drink 21 percent of our calories. That's double what it was in 1965. Our waistlines have doubled as well, not just from soda, but alcohol, fancy coffee drinks, juice, and so-called energy drinks.

I was strictly a caffeine-free Diet Coke girl, as though that made me superior. Talk about denial. My body was still a playground for soda's unwelcome chemicals, including phosphorus, which was busily leaching away the calcium from my bones.

I knew I had to kick the habit. It was a matter of health, but also one of hypocrisy. Drinking soda became harder to square with what I'd learned writing about food. You can't talk the talk when you're not walking the walk (unless, apparently, you're in public office, but that's another matter).

Being a weenie, I went for a step-down approach, the slow switch, the same kind of approach I advocate for you. For a couple of weeks, I allowed myself a soda whenever the mood struck. The caveat — I had to drink a glass of water first. That way, I figured, I'd be getting good hydration and getting in the habit of drinking more water. This turned out to be true.

It got to be that once I drank the water, I didn't want the soda.

I got down to one Diet Coke to enjoy with dinner. The rest of the day, I drank mint tea or water with a wedge of lemon for festiveness and flavor. Water became the beverage of choice, and by keeping a food journal, I discovered I'd drink anything if it was next to my computer while I was working — soda, hemlock, whatever — so it might as well be water.

Over time, the two-liter bottles of Diet Coke from my bad old days became shrouded with dust. By the time I opened one for a visiting friend, it had gone flat and fizzless.

I've been soda-free for years now and don't miss it at all. In fact, the thought of it, all sweet and foamy in my mouth, is just weird. Am I happier? Healthier? Richer? More famous? Well, I'm healthier. I have fewer colds, more stamina, glowier skin, and nails that actually grow. And I'm pretty happy. And I owe it all to literature. My own.

SOWING *the* SEEDS *of* LOVE, *or* APHRODISIACS *and* OTHER ADDITIVES

Saint Valentine was martyred sometime back in the third century, so the guy's bona fides are sketchy. The truth, as best we know, is the Romans jailed him, and while behind bars, Valentine would send word out by letter to his fans, saying buck up, all is well, don't lose heart. And thus the greeting card was born.

A couple millennia later, we in America celebrate Valentine's Day with a sharp uptick in card, rose, and chocolate sales. I will tell you this, though you may not believe me — these will not solve every romantic problem. They will not guarantee you a hookup with your obsession du jour or smooth over a rough patch with your honey. Nor is bling necessarily the answer. If it's a must-have gadget, it's obsolete already. Diamonds may be forever, but they often fund African warlords, and do you really want that on your head?

I'm a cheap date for Valentine's Day — or any day. This is, in part, why my husband, Benjamin, married me. Another reason, he says, is I have the biggest heart of anyone he knows. I think it is his nice way of saying I'm a sucker, a softie, and he is going to have to pick up the wet, gloppy chunks of my heart when it breaks yet again. I never developed a thick emotional skin. In that regard, I am like a lobster.

I never much considered the lobster (sorry, David Foster Wallace), other than noting the obvious — they are butt-ugly. (And to put such creatures in your mouths and eat them is desirable? Really?) Then I took a trip to Maine, where I learned about shedders.

From time to time, lobsters molt. Stands to reason when you think about it. If you've reached a certain size, you're going to bump up against the inside of your exoskeleton, and what then? Molt or be crushed by your very skin. So lobsters shed. Then they are still butt-ugly, on top of which they are vulnerable.

That's the downside of being in love — it turns you into a shedder. Sure, the world turns up its colors, and the secrets of the universe whisper to you and tell you how hot you are. On the other hand, your carefully constructed life splits open, crashes, and falls away. In time, you will grow another crust around yourself, but in the meantime, you are naked, bro, and out in the open waters, where anything can get you.

On the other hand, going through life with your carapace in place cuts down on your fun. So I have tried to be selective, discerning in my love interests.

I put out in the kitchen but do not do so for just anyone. I have to like you.

And you can bet the end result will be good. Or at least thought through, mused over, mentally and even physically caressed and massaged until I have the thing I feel will give you the most pleasure.

Nothing is more intimate than feeding someone. The question is, what does love taste like? What are the flavors of affection,

desire, comfort, seduction, flirtation? It depends on the one —
or ones — you're feeding. Of course it's complicated. With dinner, as with life, what we think we want isn't necessarily what we
want. Or need. The trick is divining that deeper, primal desire or
absence. That hunger.

Feeding people I love — or even like — should not be my
default. I have other talents. Being able to recite "The Love Song
of J. Alfred Prufrock" in its entirety. Pole dancing. Okay, I'm
a lousy pole dancer. But I've been feeding people since I was a
kid. My early forays into the kitchen were praised by my mother,
who'd been shooed out of the kitchen by her own mother, and
by my father, who had — and has — a sweet tooth and hoped to
cultivate a source of endless brownies. He got it.

Baking brownies for Daddy and making dinner to seduce
someone have at their root the same desire, a wish to please on a
primal level. However, the difference is ripe with possibility. This
became apparent to me at fifteen when I decided to have an orgy
for my friends.

They were seniors — two years older than me and about
twenty years more sophisticated. Except for one thing. They
talked extensively about sex but didn't have it. Oh, there was longing, all right. Some of us pined terribly for others who were, as is
the way of adolescence, clueless (about a lot of things, including,
in one case, sexual identity, but that's another story).

Um, the sex thing? I *had* had it, and with the conviction of
the newly converted, concluded it would do my friends a world
of good, too. With a terrible teen logic, I decided we should have
sex with each other. We'd be each other's initiating experience
and set each other free.

Of course, there was the lust/disinhibition issue. This group
wasn't prone to ripping off their clothes or anyone else's. Some

intervention, some assistance, was going to be necessary. So I invited everyone over for dinner. And laced the food with an aphrodisiac.

Okay, this strikes me as forty kinds of wrong now, but at the time, what I worried about was which sex stimulant and how to score it. Had I applied myself to my studies with the same determination, I'd have been valedictorian. But I was more interested in sex. In an altruistic way — you want the best for your friends.

To me, a novice recreational drug user, date-rape drugs and Spanish fly seemed both crass and iffy. However, dittany of Crete, a variety of oregano, has some historical precedent as an amatory aid, plus it has a pretty pink flower. It is, however, indigenous only to Crete. As in: Greece. As in: some six thousand miles from Miami. And me without even a driver's license yet. Dittany of Crete was not gettable in Miami back then, at least through mainstream channels and with my babysitting money. Cardamom was easier to get my hands on. Like its kin, ginger, it's a warming spice and has been warming up folks for centuries. Characters sucked on cardamom seeds in *Tales of a Thousand and One Nights*. Promising.

Even more promising, my parents would be away for the weekend. They knew my friends. Hanging out at our house and sucking everything out of the fridge is what they always did. This time, though, the eats would be different.

I took to the kitchen. I substituted regular oregano for the dittany of Crete and made — I couldn't tell you why now — a moussaka. Moussaka, that Greek mélange of layered eggplant, potatoes, zucchini, tomatoes, onions, and melting béchamel, may be classic, but it evokes a bent Greek grandmother with sensible black shoes and a whisper of a mustache. It is not sexy. Plus it requires a hell of a lot of chopping and stirring, and dirtying every pot in the kitchen. By the time I'd assembled it, I was ready to call the whole thing off. But I added a final handful of oregano and hoped for the best.

The night of the dinner, my friends arrived, innocent, unknowing, hungry. I wore a red dress which had the effect of shoving my breasts up to my chin. To paraphrase M. F. K. Fisher, I served it forth.

The moussaka was oregano-intense, all right — so much so, it had a bitter finish. But what did we know? We were teens, not food critics. Everyone ate with abandon — except for one friend who'd decided to go on a diet and left deconstructed bits of moussaka all over his plate. Too bad — of all of us, he needed to get laid the most. But big appetite or small, if the oregano was turning us on, the effect was dead subtle.

Desperate, I brought out dessert. Apple crumble. Okay, it was lacking in the looks department. It was, as crumbles are, brown and lumpy. But you couldn't miss the fragrance of the cardamom, dark, sweet, peppery. At the first bite, all talking stopped. The crumbly topping melted on the tongue (thank you, butter), the apples achieved that perfect balance of firmness and yield, with the Granny Smiths adding that soupçon of tartness to offset the sweeter Cortlands. And the cardamom — slightly honeyed, slightly dusky — struck a low note, back in the throat, deep in the viscera. It seemed to dirty-dance with our tongues.

Ahh, I thought, here we go. With cardamom, we might be on to something. I sat back, looked around, smiled, and waited.

We ate the crumble down to crumbs. But it was the only thing that got ravished. No one became touchy-feely. They did not flush, twitch, or get that happy-stupid look of hormone-revved lust. My red dress stayed on; likewise everyone else's clothes. I have never made or eaten moussaka again.

I learned my lesson — let my friends have sex in their own

time with people of their own choosing. I gave up on the idea of orgies. But not on aphrodisiacs.

The best aphrodisiac isn't in a powder or a plant; it's — eureka — in each person, something alchemical waiting to be summoned.

It took a while for me to get it right. I started in college with a guy with dark, liquid eyes and a cleft chin — the first one I ever saw on someone who wasn't Cary Grant. He had a resonant voice and a broody manner, which struck me as wildly romantic and now just seems like a pain in the ass. But I was young and foolish and smitten — smitten to the point I clamped my jaw shut every time we met, sure if I said more than hello, I would start babbling like an idiot. Perhaps he thought I was mute at first.

We circled each other for weeks, leaving vapor trails of pheromones. By this time, I'd shown myself capable of speech and potentially more. He asked me out. I countered by offering to make him dinner.

Burgers and beer would have been the safe choice, but I'm not a beer-and-burger sort of girl; and besides, that kind of food just weighs you down. Heavy was not the effect I was going for. Vegetarian but not vegan at that time, I chose cheese soufflé. Soufflés are cheap to make and so wonderfully hopeful. They inflate, they rise, they aspire. And I never had one go wrong since the first one I baked at the age of nine (I was an unusual child).

With it, I poured champagne (okay, it was cheap California *méthode champenoise* — I was on a student budget) and served a salad of soft, pale baby greens with fennel and grapefruit — pink grapefruit for that boudoir blush — dressed with a light, bright vinaigrette, the texture and acidity a nice foil for the melting unctuousness of the soufflé. For dessert, fresh raspberries. It is a meal that leaves you light. And full of longing.

Funny, I do not remember what I wore, but I remember setting the table. There were candles, of course, and flowers — daisies, not roses (again the impoverished-student issue), but they looked charming against the dark blue table linens. Blue-and-white plates made a nice contrast to the golden puff of soufflé, which, may I say, was spectacular, its crust yielding to the determined downward thrust of the serving spoon, revealing a trembling tumble of tangy, cheddary goodness within. The green salad leaves and pink grapefruit glistened with vinaigrette; slim flutes of straw-colored champagne trailed a whisper of bubbles.

Pink Grapefruit and Fennel Salad

Both grapefruit and fennel are loaded with vitamin C, antioxidants, potassium, and fiber. And walnuts are crazy with omega-3s. But what do you care about that when you just want to get laid? Well, this palate-dazzling winter salad works that angle too.

You can toss it together in a bowl, but for extra points, make a composed salad. It allows for visual seduction and is much easier than it sounds. Just mound the arugula on individual plates or a platter, scatter chopped fennel on top, and fan out the grapefruit pieces. Sprinkle with toasted nuts and freshly ground pepper.

Serves 4 to 6. Making it for a date with your potential beloved? Just halve the recipe.

1 pink grapefruit
1 fennel bulb
½ cup walnuts
¼ cup walnut oil

2 tablespoons Dijon mustard
2 tablespoons mirin
1 tablespoon agave nectar or honey
1 teaspoon fennel seeds, crushed
4 cups arugula
Freshly ground pepper

Peel the grapefruit and cut the sections into bite-size pieces. Remove and discard the seeds and trim away bitter membranes and pith. Place the grapefruit pieces in a large bowl.

Halve the fennel bulb and slice it very thinly. Add it to the grapefruit.

Preheat the oven to 350°F. Coarsely chop the walnuts and pour into a shallow baking pan. Bake until they're golden brown and have a wonderful buttery smell, about 10 minutes. Set aside to cool.

In a small bowl, whisk together the walnut oil, mustard, mirin, agave nectar, and fennel seeds. Pour the mixture over the grapefruit and fennel, toss gently, and let marinate at room temperature for 30 minutes or in the refrigerator for up to 4 hours.

Gently toss the arugula with the grapefruit and fennel. Top with the chopped walnuts and a grind or two of pepper.

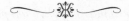

I had, alas, worked myself into such a nervous state, I was running a mild fever. It didn't hamper me any and, what the hell, gave my cheeks a bit of a glow. Gentle heat came off the candles and came off me. The white petals of the daisies fell one by one.

I could barely eat, but I didn't need to. Watching him do so was nourishment enough. The way his eyes widened with pleasure or sometimes closed told me plenty. He didn't speak much because, well, he didn't. So when it seemed appropriate, I chattered on about God knows what. Otherwise, I let him be.

Afterward, I set the crystal serving bowl brimming with tender berries on the table, no plates, no spoons. We reached in, our fingers touching by accident. Or not.

He reassessed me. He kissed me. But then he started dating this girl named Debbie, which pretty much tells you everything.

I got the menu right; I got the guy wrong.

Next on the list, a guy with naughty, twinkling eyes, a bad-boy pout, ass cheeks as taut and curved as two halves of a plum …and breath that smelled like something evil washed up in the tide. His hello, while enthusiastic, stopped me in my tracks. Rather than tell him, I fed him hillocks of tabbouleh, bright and cleansing, with parsley and mint, mesas of ginger cookies, and rivers of peppermint tea — flavors to delight the palate and neutralize the breath.

"Wonderful," he'd moan, popping another cookie in his mouth. Having grown up in a household where the only seasonings were salt and garlic powder, he'd gladly have followed me down any culinary trail. Alas, kissing him remained a problem, and I had to give him the boot.

I made another beau soup when he was ailing and presented it to him, the pot swaddled in a red-checked cloth.

"What is it?" he asked, sitting up in bed, his blue eyes bright with fever.

"Lentil soup. I made it."

"Why would you do that, baby?"

This requires explanation?

Lentils are the most easily digested of the legumes and therefore excellent for infants and those infirm or feeling off their feed.

Like their beany brothers, though, they're still protein rich. The little disks, slightly convex, not only are delightful in the mouth but inspired a whole scientific field — optics. Optical lenses get their design and name from lentils (whose botanical name is *Lens culinaris*).

Lentils require no presoaking and cook quickly, going from dried to ready to eat, bing, bang, boom. So you can make a nourishing soup with ease. Being mild tasting, they gladly take to any sort of spin. When you're feeling spirited, you can spike them with cumin and turmeric as they do in the Middle East and India (see Red Lentil Soup with Indian Spices, page 176) or with chili and mint as they do in Turkey. These flavors unlock something deliciously primal in me. But if, as with my blue-eyed love, you're in need of deep, basic comfort, simply cook the lentils with a mirepoix — finely diced celery, onions, and carrots, which act as a little bouquet for your food. Then eat. You can feel the healing course through you.

"Just taste it," I said, spooning some into his mouth.

Deep, Basic Comfort Lentil Soup

This soup is simplicity itself. I'm always tempted to embellish it with spices and vegetables, which makes it lovely but also turns it into another soup (see Red Lentil Soup with Indian Spices, page 176). Sometimes, life requires a little restraint. When it does, this is your soup.

While I normally prefer largish vegetables in my soup, here the goal is for all the vegetable bits to be roughly the same size as the lentils, hence the finer chopping.

Serves 4 to 6

1 tablespoon olive oil

2 cloves garlic, minced

4 carrots, finely chopped

3 stalks celery, finely chopped

1 cup lentils

4 cups Stone Soup (see page 84) or other vegetable broth or
    water

1 bay leaf

Sea salt and freshly ground pepper

In a large saucepan, heat the oil over medium-high heat. Add the garlic, carrots, and celery. Cook, stirring occasionally, until the vegetables are fragrant and softened, about 5 minutes.

Pick through your lentils and remove any pebbles or odd bits. Pour into the saucepan with the vegetables. Add the vegetable broth and bay leaf and bring to a boil.

Cover, reduce the heat to low, and simmer until everything has become tender and fond of each other to the point of coalescing, about 1 hour.

If a smoother, more velvety soup appeals, feel free to puree using an immersion blender, taking care to avoid splatters. Otherwise, simply season generously with salt and pepper. Feed to yourself, an invalid, an infant, or anyone who needs more from less.

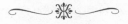

Blue Eyes improved quickly. Our relationship did not. A man with no appreciation for homemade lentil soup will have no appreciation for the kind of person who makes it.

The intensity, inexperience, and angst of youth are, happily, behind me. The angst of adulthood, alas, is not. But still, if I meet you and I like you, I want to cook for you, to feed you what best satisfies your own particular hunger. I can't help it.

It seemed to me perfectly natural at the end of interviewing a Pulitzer-nominated novelist, to invite the man to dinner. Along with his wife and two young children. It was only a few days later that it dawned on me — I did not know these people, I had not met these people. And vice versa. This novelist is famous and acclaimed — what would he want with me? And now he and his entire family were coming to our house to eat. What the hell was I thinking? But plans were already under way, and besides, I had already concocted a menu too good to miss: champagne, kalamatas, pistachios, and toasted pita with Greek pea spread to start; moving on to fig, fennel, and arugula salad, served with a paella — fish-free, made with vegetables and quinoa and scented with a dizzying amount of saffron — and a lusty zinfandel; and for dessert, almond cake with roasted pears and a golden Sauternes. All served by a cook whose only desire was to please.

The pleasure, it turns out, was mine. Good food, good wine — they help an evening along. Dazzling, charming company like the author and his family helps, too. But that's nothing you can count on.

You don't have to be famous to be at my table. You don't even have to be human. I did the same thing when I babysat a friend's pet rabbit, preparing a feast of shaved carrots, a few raisins, and tender celery leaves. The raisins were well received, but rabbits are easy. People are the puzzle and altogether harder to woo.

Unconventional but Seductive Veggie Paella

Paella, Spain's iconic dish, is traditionally made with rice, meat, fowl, and/or seafood. I've substituted quicker-cooking, higher-protein quinoa for the rice and lighter, brighter veggies for the animal bits. But I've left some tradition intact. As with true, classic paella, this vegetarian version is heady with saffron and feeds a crowd.

Serves 6 to 8

1 mild dried chili, such as ancho
4 tablespoons olive oil
6 cloves garlic, chopped
1 tablespoon sweet or smoked paprika
Generous pinch of saffron
One 15-ounce can diced tomatoes
4 carrots, chopped
1 fennel bulb, chopped
1 bunch scallions or 1 spring onion, chopped
8 ounces mushrooms, sliced
4 cups Stone Soup (see page 84) or other vegetable broth or
    water
2 cups quinoa, rinsed
Sea salt and freshly ground pepper
One 15-ounce can artichoke hearts, rinsed, drained, and
    quartered
2 roasted red bell peppers (jarred are fine), cut into strips
12 cherry or grape tomatoes, halved if large
Chopped fresh flat-leaf parsley for garnish
Fennel fronds for garnish

In a small bowl, soak the chili in enough hot water to cover until softened, about 20 minutes. Drain the chili and chop.

In a large, deep skillet or Spanish cazuela, heat 2 tablespoons of the olive oil over medium heat. Add the chopped chili and garlic. Cook, stirring occasionally, until the garlic turns golden, 4 to 5 minutes. Add the paprika, the saffron, and the canned tomatoes and their juice. Cook, stirring occasionally, until thick and fragrant, about 2 minutes.

Transfer to a blender or food processor, and puree until smooth, about 1 minute.

No need to clean the skillet. Use it to heat the remaining 2 tablespoons olive oil over medium-high heat. Add the carrots, fennel, and scallions. Cook, stirring occasionally, until the vegetables relax and are gilded with oil, about 5 minutes. Add the mushrooms and cook until the mushrooms darken and become tender, another 5 minutes. Return the chili-tomato sauce to the skillet and stir to combine. Add 1 cup of the vegetable broth and stir for just a few minutes, until a thickish sauce forms.

Add the quinoa and an additional 1 cup broth to the skillet. Stir gently, reduce the heat to medium, and cook without stirring, rotating the skillet occasionally to distribute the heat evenly. After 10 minutes, add the remaining 2 cups broth and cook until all the liquid is absorbed and the quinoa grains have popped and expanded, about 10 minutes. Taste and give it a good seasoning of sea salt and freshly ground pepper.

Gently press the artichoke hearts, red bell pepper strips, and cherry tomatoes into the top of the paella. Be artsy. Remove the paella pan from the heat and cover with a lid or wrap tightly with aluminum foil. Let rest for 10 to 15 minutes.

Garnish with parsley and feathery fennel fronds.

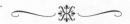

Experience has taught me coaxing out someone's inner aphrodisiac means coupling the familiar with the exotic — scenting
homey apple crumble with earthy cardamom, leavening a typi-
cally heavy meal with an ethereal soufflé. It means giving someone the welcome of the known, but giving it a twist, so you taste
something familiar in a whole new way. It is discovery, it is revelation, it is like falling in love with what you already know. Having
a warm heart in the kitchen counts, too. Seduction in the bedroom
or the kitchen is harder when you're feeling pissy.

In some ways, I still cook to seduce. Or please. Or comfort. I'm
a married woman, after all. Benjamin eats what I cook every day
and loves what I feed him, whether it's lentil soup or cardamom-
scented apple crumble or ripe, naked berries. This is not why I
married him. But it's nice.

I still love cardamom and add it to dishes from curries to
crumbles. Because you never know.

Amorous Cardamom Apple Crumble

*Admit it, you were waiting for this recipe. It's wonderful eaten warm and
naked, by you and your love, clothing optional.*

**Serves 6 to 8 — or 2 very turned-on people with lots of
leftovers**

Oil for the pie pan
¾ cup plus 2 tablespoons unbleached all-purpose flour
¾ cup old-fashioned oats (also known as rolled oats)
1½ cups brown sugar

Zest and juice of 1 lemon

2½ teaspoons ground cardamom

½ cup (1 stick) vegan margarine, such as Earth Balance,
    softened

6 apples, preferably a combination of tart and sweet, peeled
    and sliced

1 teaspoon ground cinnamon

Preheat the oven to 375°F. Lightly oil a 9-inch pie pan.

In a medium bowl, combine ¾ cup of the flour, the oats, ¾ cup of the brown sugar, the lemon zest, and 1½ teaspoons of the cardamom. Stir together until the mixture is combined. Work in the vegan margarine until the mixture just turns into a crumble. A food processor can do the job in less than a minute — be careful not to overmix. Using a wooden mixing spoon gives you greater crumb control and lets you put extra heart into it — it'll take a couple minutes. Set the crumb mixture aside.

Put the apple slices in a large bowl, pour the lemon juice over all, and toss together. Add the remaining ¾ cup brown sugar, the remaining 2 tablespoons flour, the remaining 1 teaspoon cardamom, and the cinnamon. Stir gently until just combined.

Fill the pie pan with the apples and top with the crumble mixture, lightly packing the crumbs on top. Bake for 30 to 45 minutes, or until the crumble is bubbling, golden brown, and fragrant as hell.

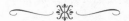

GENTLE NUDGE *the* THIRD: DUMPING *the* DUDS

Our relationship with food is a metaphor. It reflects our relationship with everything else. Nasty food habits, toxic life decisions. If you're treating your body — your fabulous, one-of-a-kind body

— like trash, how are you treating your family? Your friends? Your community? Your planet?

A bad food relationship is just as awful as a bad romantic relationship. You meet someone, it starts out great, violins, fireworks, hot sex. Then comes the letdown. Turns out Mr. Wonderful has an irritating habit of breaking dates, an interfering mother with whom he currently lives, and a somewhat unresolved relationship with his ex.

Maybe you cut him some slack at first, because that's the kind of person you are. But come on, how many times are you going to be taken in by some fool offering you that grin that's not as disarming as he'd like to believe, along with the pretty promise that this time things will be different, baby? (Not that I'm speaking from experience or anything.) You wouldn't keep dating a loser, darling. So ditch him.

Alas, taking away someone or something we love — even when we know it's bad for us — stinks. Of course, we all know this on some level, but our dog taught me the lesson all over again when, in her naughty puppy days, she chewed off the head of her favorite plush toy. As I preferred her not to eat wads of cotton stuffing, I tried to take it away from her. Bad idea. Growling and snapping ensued.

Deprivation may make saints of some, but it makes the rest of us mean, small, creepy, and generally unpleasant. Plus it doesn't work. Take away our toy, and we will turn to something else. Your shoe, perhaps.

So what does work? Slow, gentle change and a little distraction. The only way I could extract the mauled dog toy without being savaged was to offer her something else. Look! For you! Pretty new toy. Nice doggie.

Can't live without ice cream? Enjoy it. But try eating just a spoonful or two less than you did last night. Serve it to yourself in something pretty; you deserve it, babe. Then when you're out of ice cream, don't buy more. What the eye can't see, the heart don't grieve, as an Aussie sweetie told me once. Breathe. You don't have to commit to doing this forever; just try it now, just get through now. Distract yourself. Coconut milk ice cream, frozen yogurt, and pure fruit sorbet are luscious and offer less fat and fewer calories than ice cream. Pretty new toys can be good for you, too.

Not only will you have dumped a bad habit — a major coup — you'll be creating a positive new one. There's neurological evidence that repetition of new behavior can rewire a scrambled brain. Even yours. Once you pave the way for new neurocircuitry, it seems to green-light other changes that once seemed impossible. Think of it as psychospiritual feng shui.

Getting rid of duds, whether dietary or live-in, takes time, patience, and the absolute and abundant belief that you deserve better. And you do. You deserve to be the healthiest, hottest, most joyful you possible. You may find over time you can ditch your old dud of an ice cream fix and feel terrific about yourself besides. Häagen-Dazs may suffer, but you won't.

Chapter

2 *the* FLOWERING

We think of flowers as pretty. Nature wants us to, arranging them in pleasing, symmetrical shapes and decorating them in a whole mad paint box of colors, from the gentle lavender pastels of water lilies captured by Monet, to ginger's red-and-orange in-your-face spikes and spires, which inspired Gauguin. If you've never evolved beyond the simple five-petal-flower-drawing stage, you're still in luck. Loving flowers has nothing to do with artistic talent. It's how we're hardwired. Because botanically speaking, they are the sex organs of plants.

Blooming flowers gladden our hearts after a cold, gray winter, but their main agenda is to attract birds and insects, to stimulate pollination and get life's party going. While the flowers pop their saucy heads out of the cold earth, the sap rises in young trees. And in all species. Spring is libidinous, fecund, fun. In spring, as Alfred, Lord Tennyson wrote in "Locksley Hall," "a livelier iris changes on the burnish'd dove; / In the Spring a young man's fancy lightly turns to thoughts of love." This is a decorous,

Victorian way of saying in the spring, we feel the love. We feel the lust. All life forms come out of dormancy, and we're strutting our stuff.

Maybe not all of us. April is the cruelest month, according to T. S. Eliot (breathe — this is our last poetry reference for a while). What Eliot meant by this is that April can be a con. It's supposed to be the month in which everything comes into flower. But then it snows. Or you wipe out walking the path that was so firm beneath your feet yesterday but that has, thanks to the spring thaw, morphed into a mud bath from which your dignity and your Jimmy Choos will never recover. It's supposed to be spring. But you're still swaddled in sweaters and can't kick the sinus infection you got back in January. Maybe the weather is delightful. The sun is out, the lilacs are in full, audacious bloom, their fragrance cloying, pervasive, and migraine inducing, and everyone is pairing up and going at it, including your ex. The two of you just broke up, but he hasn't been pining. In fact, he's getting married (to someone else), so you're just a mite hard-pressed to see the glory in everything, all right? So just back the hell off.

Buck up. Spring happens once a year, but even without climate change, the rules are different for humankind. You are not an annual, one that grows, flowers, shoots its seed, so to speak, and dies. No, the really great thing about our species is we can come into flower again and again. It is a coming into self, a blooming, a sense of realizing the extent of our own incredible talents and powers.

Say you've been in a holding pattern; a not-good-but-not-bad treading-water phase. Then one morning, you awake and delight to the trill of the sparrow that's been singing its heart out for weeks, only you're just now hearing it. You find your footing in a previously rocky relationship or at last figure out how not to crash the office's new software system. The scales fall from your eyes; the numbers drop from your bathroom scale; your musk is in the air; your very presence seems to charge the ions around you; the gods beam down and rain prizes and presents upon you. Or at least you think, okay, maybe this has all been to the good, after all. And though it's nothing you might bring up in your carpool, you feel your soul lift and lighten. You feel joy. Flowering is when life tells you *yes*.

For me, sex is the best yes out there, any time of the year. I am a nice, married woman, but even so, desire can surprise and awaken you in odd, unpredictable spurts. I'm not talking about erectile dysfunction drugs; I'm talking about when attraction floods you for no reason, like suddenly getting a crazy-ass crush on the organic farmer at the local farmers' market or that senator with the weird hair. It gives you a reason to smile through your committee meeting, wear lipstick, or get a haircut. It does not always coincide with the season, and hallelujah for that — I'd hate to think love as we know it has to be stuffed in between April and June, or else we're out of luck for another year. It can happen in your own spring and well beyond, too, even when you're older and supposedly wiser. Desire makes happy suckers of us all and makes us blossom into creations both beautiful and vulnerable.

You deserve flowers. They belong in your life. And in your diet. Orange blossom, lavender, jasmine, and rose are a few with terrific culinary applications, adding their haunting fragrance to food and drinks, along with a whisper of other lands and definite healthful properties. If this sounds weird, let's start with a super-basic herbal concoction, what the French call a tisane, or infusion — a cup of lavender tea.

Lavender Tea

Lavender infusion is pale but has a surprisingly bracing flavor. It's just a wee bit soapy tasting. That means it's cleansing. Good. It'll wash those old negative feelings right out of you. Breathe. Feel the tea work its magic. Let it soothe you; let it heal your heart.

Makes a generous pot, serving 1 to 4

2 teaspoons lavender buds[*]

Put on a kettle of water and bring to a boil.

Fill a tea infuser with lavender buds; put the infuser in a teapot. Pour in the boiling water. Let steep for about 3 minutes.

You may pour it into a mug, but it would be happiest — and so would you — if you served it in your grandmother's china teacup, the one with all the flowers on it.

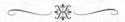

You've probably eaten other flowers, the flowering parts of plants, without causing a scene, without even realizing it. Chili pepper, without which I would not care to live, qualifies. So do goji berries, the superfruit of the moment, as well as peas, cucumbers, and many of your nightshade vegetables, including peppers, tomatoes, and eggplant. If only David, my late father-in-law, had known eggplant is a sex organ, he might have been more inclined to eat it.

---

[*]   Available in many culinary shops and a bazillion places online.

Down and Dirty Rice

What makes traditional New Orleans dirty rice dirty is the addition of what James Joyce described in Ulysses *as "the inner organs of beasts and fowl" — gizzards. Um, no thanks. Chopped eggplant — the flowering, sexual part of the plant — takes the place of organ meat in this supersatisfying veggie version. It's nice on one of those surprisingly chilly spring nights. The dish is not too spicy but you can make it that way. That's what Tabasco sauce is for. It's made from Louisiana's Tabasco chili, which is also a flowering vegetable.*

Serves 6 to 8

5 cups Stone Soup (see page 84) or other vegetable broth or
    water
1½ cups rice (white is traditional, brown is more
    healthful)
1 bay leaf
1 tablespoon olive oil
6 cloves garlic, chopped
1 large onion, chopped
1 medium eggplant, chopped
2 stalks celery, chopped
1 green bell pepper, chopped
2 tomatoes, chopped, or one 15-ounce can diced tomatoes
2 teaspoons sweet paprika
1 handful fresh thyme leaves or 1 teaspoon dried thyme
Sea salt and freshly ground pepper
Juice of 1 lemon
1 bunch fresh flat-leaf parsley, chopped
1 cup cooked edamame (optional)

In a large pot, bring 3 cups of the broth to a boil over high heat. Add the rice and bay leaf. Stir gently, cover, and reduce the heat to low. Simmer until all the liquid is absorbed and the rice is tender, about 30 minutes for white rice, 40 minutes for brown rice. Remove the bay leaf and set the rice aside. (The rice can be stored in an airtight container in the refrigerator for a day or two; bring to room temperature before proceeding with the recipe.)

In a large skillet, heat the oil over medium-high heat. Add the garlic, onion, and eggplant. Cook, stirring occasionally, until the vegetables soften, about 5 minutes. Add the celery, green bell pepper, tomatoes, paprika, and thyme. Continue cooking, giving the vegetables a stir now and again, until they are tender and gilded with oil and spices, 5 to 8 minutes. Stir in the cooked rice and the remaining 2 cups broth.

Reduce the heat to medium and cook until all the liquid is absorbed yet the mixture is still moist, about 10 minutes.

Season with salt and pepper. Stir in the lemon juice and parsley. For a pop of protein and bright green color, fold in the edamame, if you like.

This will keep covered for several days in the fridge, and the flavor improves over time.

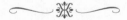

STANDING *on* CEREMONY

The big lessons, from seasonal eating to eating together as a family, are a little like sex. It's all well and good to hear about, but it can seem like the practice or politics in another country — very far removed from your own overstuffed life. It's only when you experience it yourself that you get that sense of wow, where have I been all these years? May the delights and mysteries of the world reveal themselves to you in the first go. However, most of us need to lather, rinse, and repeat these lessons over and over again before the grin-making, grateful-to-be-alive feeling or the "Ah, now I get it" feeling sinks in. This is the nature of imprinting for us imperfect beings. So whether you're instructing or learning, it helps to come to the big lessons with patience. Because it's always going to be somebody's first time. And you want it to be fabulous.

My family steeped me in ritual before I even knew it — stealth induction, very clever. Friday nights, we'd go to the home of Marcella and her husband, my grandfather. His name was Aaron, but he was not the sort of guy I'd dream of calling by his first name. Ever. Even Benjamin, who was twenty-five when he met him, referred to him as Mr. Kanner, and may I say, his voice occasionally broke when he did so.

The chummiest I got was to call him Grandpa. He didn't notice me most of the time, and I tried to encourage that by keeping the hell out of his way. We were related and yet like different species to each other. He was not kid friendly, nor was his house, all stone and formal upholstered furniture and breakable objets d'art.

There were no toys on hand, just one well-worn copy of *The Velveteen Rabbit*, which I dutifully read every Friday, since my cousins weren't interested. We were — *are* — close in age, so when we weren't busy fighting, we played together, chasing each other down the hall, our shrieks ringing out; and though we were told to be careful, I wiped out on the living-room terrazzo and knocked out my front tooth. It was only a baby tooth, so no harm done, other than initial trauma and profuse bleeding everywhere. Just another Friday evening, another walk along the knife edge between order and chaos, a chaos just held in check by dinner.

We sat at the dinner table together, the whole family — that

was just the deal. By the time I was in the picture, the whole family meant Aaron, Marcella, their two grown sons, their wives, five
grandchildren, and at least one family friend or distant cousin
or someone my grandmother had run into and invited, as well.
We crowded around the table — Italian, midcentury, with all its
leaves in — my grandparents presiding at either end, me usually
squished in between adults, straddling a table leg.

My grandparents weren't observant Jews, but even so, Friday
night, Sabbath, was special. The table would be set with starched
white linen, the kind you never see anymore, sterling, china, and
crystal stemware.

Dinner would mean soup or salad to start; a serious main
course, which might be roast leg of lamb or stuffed peppers or
spaghetti and meatballs; rolls and butter; potato or rice. There
were vegetables, but of a distinctly old-school style, lacking
brightness, flavor, freshness, and oomph. In regular rotation —
peas and carrots (frozen and then boiled) and gelid iceberg lettuce
salads. There were marinated artichoke hearts, which I came to
love once I realized their name had nothing to do with choking
your heart, and asparagus, canned, anemic, slimy, and, we were
told, "a delicacy." Like that would make us want to eat it.

On the bright side, there was dessert. Marcella was gifted in
the ways of lemon Bundt cakes, coconut layer cakes, brownies,
sugar cookies, and buttery, ground-almond cookies rolled in a
profligate amount of powdered sugar. She called them wedding
cookies, but they're beloved all over, with many iterations —
they're called Mexican wedding cakes, Greek kourabiedes, and
ghraybeh across the Middle East. My favorite name for them is
liar's cookies, because as soon as you bite into one, you're dusted
and incriminated. Or worse. I could never manage to eat one
without inhaling the powdered sugar and having a coughing fit.

The rest of the meal, though, was prepared by Cora, my grandparents' magnificent housekeeper. She was large, elderly, motherly, black, but with the heart and sensibility of a yenta. Cora had a definitive sense of How Things Ought to Be that I can only wonder at. The Friday night family dinner edict may well have come from her.

She cooked for all of us, including those of us too young to realize what a big honking deal it is to prepare enormous multicourse meals for a horde. Also a big honking deal — exposing little kids to grown-up food. Very grown-up. Archaic, even — I mean, whose idea was beef tongue? Who thought it would be a big seller to a six-year-old? Cooking it with raisins might have lent it sweetness, but it looked like what it was, with all those weird little papillae bumps on it. Don't get me started.

If we didn't love the tongue, there were no McNugget backups. We could eat or not eat what was being served; there were plenty of other things on the table; and well, better luck next Friday — maybe there'd be fried chicken.

I'm sure there were more than a few meltdowns, maybe from the kids, maybe from their parents. I have a vague but recurring memory of Cora threatening to kill herself if we didn't eat the mashed potatoes and my grandfather getting up from the table to pour himself a tumbler of scotch.

Maybe he wasn't so old, but he had all the accoutrements: false teeth, which he kept in a glass by the bed, hearing aid, thick glasses, and — yecchh — a truss. The precursor to the more macho weight belt, this was a complicated, allegedly flesh-colored, many-strapped thing that mostly resided on a chintz bedroom chair, where its sole purpose seemed to be to scare the bejesus out of me. I gave it a wide berth, never so much as touched it.

What with the truss and my debacle on the terrazzo, the

kitchen became my playroom of choice. I was obsessed by the big, black gas range with a cooktop that lit up witchy rings of blue flame. Marcella and Cora's knives worked better as bludgeons than as sharp implements, so I couldn't do too much damage. The two women didn't mind having me underfoot, but they had dinner to make and went about their business. They didn't talk about process or recipes; both had experience and instinct. And perhaps in Cora's case, recipes were her source of power, and she wasn't about to give that up.

If they weren't instructive, they weren't restrictive, either, especially my grandmother. If six-year-old Ellen wanted to dump a box of raisins in the brownie batter, she was all for it. The kitchen was where I had my first sense of *Yes*, where I caught a glimpse of the self I still want to be the rest of the time — clever, creative, composed, not tripping up on my own craziness.

But you can't stay in the kitchen forever. Cora died, leaving my grandparents stranded and clueless. They hired and fired a series of housekeepers, all of whom were doomed because they weren't Cora.

Marcella tried to keep the Friday evenings going, but she and my grandfather were well and properly old by then. The granddaughters were older, too, and suddenly fuggy with teenage girl hormones. We served the food, whisked away the plates (sometimes before people had finished eating), and cleaned up, but we had school and social things and other interests. We had Friday-night dates with boys. Even when we managed to show up at our grandparents' house, we were so goofy and moody, my grandfather must have yearned for the past, when we were smaller and more tractable.

Looking back, I'm appalled by how casually we, the grandchildren, took things. We assumed Friday night meant it was time to trot out the heavy table linens; that was how the world worked. We shattered more than a few of those crystal glasses. But now I think it's not such a bad thing to have the line blurred between ceremony and daily life, to fold one into the other. That's how I like to live.

Benjamin and I eat dinner together, no matter how late we've worked or how crappy the day might have been. It may not be posh, but it'll be home cooked and crazy with whatever's in season. We use Marcella's sterling silverware — we never did get around to buying stainless — and plates we got in Kappabashi, Tokyo's restaurant district. They're heavy, blue-and-white, each different but all painted with scenes of old Japan — boys chasing butterflies, a tree bent by the wind, a dragon reaching out a claw. The table is lit with tapers in tall brass candlesticks that, along with the silver, could use a bit of polish.

Now is when we share our respective days, our dreams, our deadlines, the lyrics to that song Benjamin just downloaded, and my idea for a great thing to do with barley. With it, we usually share a glass of wine. It returns us to ourselves.

After dinner, Benjamin and I often move to the living room, a riot of Marrakech red and Caribbean blue, with pieces from all the places we've been to and loved. We recline on the low Moroccan couch, facing each other like bookends, the soles of our feet just touching if I stretch.

It is an epic couch that can seat many friends who come over to laugh and drink and eat. If they sometimes fall asleep there, too, we try to take this not as an insult, but as a sort of compliment — that you're welcome here; you can be who you are; and if at the moment you are sleepy or tiddly, then you nap, and we will tuck a quilt around you and try to whisper and keep the dog from licking your face. And when you wake up, the party will resume, we will be glad to see you all over again, and there will be something wonderful to eat.

Farinata

In Liguria, they call it farinata; in Provence, they call it socca. Because this Mediterranean pancake is made with chickpea flour, it's not just luscious, it's gluten-free. With a crispy crust and a tender inside, it's great by itself, or topped with roasted vegetables, tapenade, sweet and tangy jewel-tone Red Onion Jam (page 63), or vibrant Spring Pea Puree (page 64). You can make the batter ahead and bung the frittata in the oven, enjoy a glass of wine, and your farinata will be crisp, hot, and ready to serve.

Take it from stylish appetizer to more of a meal by serving it with a harvest of fresh roasted vegetables or a big, tumbling kale salad.

Serves 4

1 cup chickpea flour*
¾ cup water plus 1 tablespoon
¼ cup olive oil, plus more for the skillet
Sea salt and freshly ground pepper

Pour the chickpea flour into a medium bowl. Slowly pour in the water, stirring constantly, until a thick batter forms. Add the ¼ cup olive oil and stir until just combined. Cover and refrigerate for at

---

* Chickpea flour is available in some natural food stores and in Middle Eastern markets, where it's sometimes called besan.

least 1 hour and up to overnight. The batter should be creamy and golden, with texture and color like tahini's.

Place one rack in the uppermost position of the oven and another rack in the middle position. Preheat the broiler. Lightly oil an 8- or 9-inch skillet.

Pour the batter into the skillet, using a spatula to spread the mixture into an even layer. Sprinkle salt and pepper on top.

Place the skillet on the uppermost rack and broil until the farinata is golden, starts to firm up, and takes on a pancake appearance, 8 to 10 minutes.

Turn off the broiler and set the oven to 450°F. Transfer the farinata to the middle rack. Bake until the farinata smells toasty and a light brown crust forms on top, about 10 minutes.

Remove from oven and let cool slightly. Slice into wedges and serve.

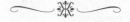

Red Onion Jam

This tangy onion jam is good with farinata or flatbread or dolloped on any grain or legume salad, and fabulous with fresh, ripe tomatoes.

Makes about 2 cups

2 red onions, halved
1 tablespoon olive oil
1 cup cabernet or other red wine
¼ cup agave nectar or honey

2 tablespoons balsamic vinegar
1 handful fresh thyme leaves
Sea salt and freshly ground pepper

Slice the onion halves thinly, so the slices form half-moons. Very stylish.

In a large skillet, heat the oil over medium-high heat. Add the onions and cook, stirring occasionally, until the onions soften and turn translucent, about 10 minutes. Add the wine, agave nectar, balsamic vinegar, and thyme, and cook, uncovered, until the liquid reduces and turns garnet colored and syrupy, about 10 minutes. Keep stirring as the mixture reduces, to keep the onions from sticking to the bottom of the pan.

Cover the skillet, reduce the heat to low, and cook until the mixture becomes jammy, about 15 minutes. Let cool. Season with salt and pepper.

The onion jam can be stored in an airtight container in the refrigerator for up to 2 weeks.

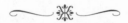

Spring Pea Puree

This puree is easy, bright in color, thanks to the peas and mint, bright in palate, thanks to the lemon and mint. Two juicy lemons should give you all the juice you need. Sometimes, though, life hands you pithy lemons, in which case a third lemon may be necessary.

Makes 1¼ cups

1½ cups fresh or frozen peas, thawed
1 clove garlic
1 bunch fresh mint
Juice of 2 or 3 lemons
¼ cup olive oil
Sea salt

Blitz the peas, garlic, mint, lemon juice, and olive oil in a food processor until smooth and well combined, about 2 minutes. Taste and season with salt.

The puree can be stored in an airtight container in the refrigerator for several days.

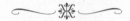

I'd like to think I'm just naturally brilliant and generous that way, but it's all due to imprinting. Over more than a few Friday nights, both Cora and Marcella inadvertently instilled in me an antipathy toward eating animals, but they also gave me the sense that a shared meal is both party and social cement — the thing that brings us together and keeps us together. And of course, it has to be beautiful. You honor your guests, whether they're kings or cousins, whether they're seven or seventy.

(Note to self: polish the silver and candlesticks.)

This belief, this practice, is my True Religion without it being, you know, true religion. Or maybe it is the truest religion. Long before it was a career path, hospitality was a moral imperative for all faiths. Inns and guesthouses had yet to dot the landscape. Airplanes wouldn't be invented for centuries. If you wanted to get somewhere, you walked. Or if you were part of the 1 percent, perhaps you had a mule or horse or camel.

There was no heading to Disneyland; you were on the Silk Route for trade or making a religious pilgrimage. On foot. And if you got a little tired or peckish on the road, you prayed someone would take you in. And if they had you bunk with the sheep or gave you their bread when, please, you're gluten intolerant, you didn't have a lot of recourse. You couldn't post a rant on TripAdvisor. So you were grateful for what you got, and it really brought home the Golden Rule.

Okay, things are a little different today. We outsource hospitality. And charge for it. So you can get things the way you want them. And yet, we've lost something, that desire, or at least that willingness, to open our homes and hearts. It means putting it out there, letting your guard down a little. In Buddhism it's known as *dana*, or generosity, but more than being generous, it's *wanting* to be generous.

I'm no more Buddhist than I am any other religion, but as a precept, *dana*'s a keeper. In the same way I have no problem mixing it up in the kitchen, I cherry-pick bits from different faiths. This is a no-no among the hard-core religious and probably offends everyone.

But people do it all the time. I mean, look at the Bible. If you want to find justification for any sort of behavior, it's in there. It's just a matter of interpretation. Including what a supreme being had in mind for us to eat. If you think there's a line in the sand between Jews and Christians or Democrats and Republicans, the difference between omnivores/meat eaters and vegetarians/vegans/meatless folks is a mile-wide chasm. And, of course, both sides think they're right.

In Genesis 1:29, the word, as Adam and Eve got it, was, "Behold, I have given you every plant yielding seed that is on the face of all the earth, and every tree with seed in its fruit. You shall have them for food." You can read that and conclude God wants us to be meatless.

Then you can read Genesis 9:3, in which God tells Noah, "Every moving thing that liveth shall be meat for you; even as the green herb have I given you all things," and conclude God's given us the okay to eat animals.

Or you can reckon, as I do, that Noah was a whiner. That he yammered and yammered and said, "But I don't like seeds and herbs. And we're stuck here in the rain on this stupid boat, and I'm hungry." God just gave in and said, all right, already, eat what you like; let it be on your head.

I'm a little skeptical about Peter, who in Acts 10:9–15 hears a voice telling him nothing is forbidden him to eat. Some religious pros believe the voice to be God's, but we weren't there. Who knows? Maybe Peter was just crazed with hunger and suffering auditory hallucinations.

So we go back to Genesis 1:28, the bit where the Lord gave man dominion over all the animals.

Yes, but that doesn't say we should eat them, too. Dominion is not the same as domination. I prefer to think the interpretation here is: we are custodians of our fellow animals, and since we have this fairly well-developed cerebral cortex that puts us in charge, it's our job to look after them. With compassion, not cruelty. And without making them for dinner.

Those made nervous by a meatless diet like to cite Romans 14:2, which says, "The weak person eats only vegetables." And though I've read an interpretation saying, oh, the Bible doesn't really mean it, even I've got to say that sounds pretty definitive. But then the scripture reads, "Let not the one who eats despise the one who abstains, and let not the one who abstains pass judgment on the one who eats, for God has welcomed him" (Romans 14:3).

And there's 1 Corinthians 8:8, which says, "Meat commendeth us not to God."

I am amazed by how many biblical references I know, considering I'm a heathen. But I had enough Sunday school before dropping out to know according to the Good Book, God laid down a scant few rules — ten of 'em. We have a hard enough time following these (some kind of human design flaw). How many elected officials alone have skirted or shrugged off three of your basic commandments — thou shalt not lie, thou shalt not steal, thou shalt not commit adultery?

So am I questioning God? No. I'm questioning us. Because while the message might be a little confusing, basically God says we can choose what we eat. The question becomes, what do we choose?

I choose compassion, toward animals of all kinds. Including — though it's sometimes a struggle — my own kind, the human kind. Which brings me to one of my biblical faves, Proverbs 15:17 — "Better is a dinner of herbs where love is than a fattened ox and hatred with it."

The way I interpret the Bible is the way I choose to live — with a supersized portion of compassion, hold the meat, hold the side of hatred.

My issue with formal religion is my issue with government. The guys at the top may go into the job with all the good intentions in the world, but once in power, they get a little too cocky. The tenets of religion get to be like a bill in Congress — there's some good bits in there you can get behind, but they're bundled with other things you cannot in good faith espouse but are forced to go along with anyway. That just doesn't feed me.

Another thing: many formal religions have used — or skewed — the tenets of their faith to justify bloody bits. You know, the

Crucifixion, the Spanish Inquisition, the slaying of the firstborn, jihad, stuff like that. With that comes the sense of we're right and you're wrong. Centuries upon centuries of it, and we still haven't realized it doesn't work.

I bypass all that breast-beating-and-bloodshed-in-the-name-of-God stuff. There's a reason Easter and Passover come in spring — at their heart, they honor seasonal renewal. Well, we can all celebrate that, and while we're at it, let's celebrate Rongali Bihu, otherwise known as Assamese New Year, the mid-April holiday when the northeast part of India marks the coming of spring. The festivities go on all week long, and how can you not love a holiday where cows are groomed and festooned with flowers?

At all the spring holidays, we gather to share ritual foods, the most direct route to season and spirit. We literally take it in. Food is the way we connect; it is the lens through which we see the world. It is creation, it is re-creation, it is nurturing, it is hope.

Judeo-Christian Biblical Barley and Herb Salad

This barley salad has life force and history. Cheap, fortifying, and loaded with fiber, barley feeds five thousand people in the Book of John and is a hit in the Old Testament, too. These days, most people consider barley — if they consider it at all — as something wintery, perhaps sharing space with mushrooms in a warming bowl of soup. Here, this ancient whole grain gets the tabbouleh treatment and becomes a significant salad loaded with herbs (and love — see Proverbs quote above).

Nice as part of a biblical meze (Middle Eastern tapas, if you will), served alongside a blob of hummus and flatbread or with roasted eggplant, it's just right for spring.

Tahini is an extremely luscious sesame paste, available in Middle Eastern groceries, natural food stores, and most supermarkets. Like natural (preservative-free) peanut butter, tahini tends to separate, with the oil floating to the top of the sesame goodness below. Stir well before using.

Serves 4 to 6

2 cups Stone Soup (see page 84) or other vegetable broth or
   water
1 cup barley
1 bunch fresh mint, chopped
1 bunch fresh cilantro, chopped
1 bunch fresh flat-leaf parsley, chopped
3 scallions, chopped
1 tomato, chopped
Juice of 1 lemon
2 tablespoons olive oil
1 teaspoon ground cumin
Pinch of red pepper flakes
½ teaspoon agave nectar or honey
1 handful kalamata olives, pitted
2 tablespoons tahini
Sea salt and freshly ground pepper

In a large pot, bring the vegetable broth to a boil over high heat. Add the barley. Cover, reduce the heat to low, and simmer until the liquid is absorbed and the grains are tender, about 30 minutes.

Fluff the cooked barley with a fork and set aside to cool. (The cooked barley can be stored in an airtight container in the refrigerator for a day or two; bring to room temperature before proceeding with the recipe.) Stir in the herbs, scallions, and tomato.

In a small bowl, whisk together the lemon juice, olive oil,

cumin, red pepper flakes, and agave nectar. Pour over the barley and stir until the grains are evenly coated with the dressing. Stir in the kalamatas.

Refrigerate in an airtight container for at least 2 hours. The dressing will soften and moisten the barley.

Remove the barley salad from the refrigerator. Drizzle the tahini over the barley salad and season with salt and pepper. The kalamatas add some saltiness of their own, so don't season until just before serving.

Serve cool or at room temperature.

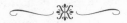

KEEPING *the* FAITH

I used to think I was rejecting my faith. Mostly, I was rejecting gefilte fish. Although not part of the true Passover plate, it has somehow become a holiday tradition in many families, including, alas, mine. You could call gefilte fish by its French name, *quenelles de poisson*, but in any language, it is minced fish shaped into dumplings and poached. I call it a fish ball, and it still makes me panicky. It is pale and lifeless, where I crave color; mushy, where I crave crunch. Wet, with disturbing gelatinous bits adhering to it, it slides all over the plate despite the sprigs of parsley or dill often used to garnish and brighten it up and perhaps serve as an anchor. I did not become vegan in order to get a gefilte fish reprieve. But it's a nice side benefit.

And yet gefilte fish is, for some, the taste of home. I understand that primal pull. Fine, you can have mine. You can have all the Ashkenazic food of Central Europe, the food of my childhood holidays. The brisket, the blintzes, the boiled, the bland. It's a cuisine that makes more sense in Minsk than Miami.

The soft, bright, cleansing mint, the tart spritz of lemon, and the oily, inky, salty kalamatas in the Judeo-Christian Biblical Barley and Herb Salad are the flavors of Sephardic cuisine, the cuisine of the Jews of Morocco, the Middle East, and the Mediterranean. Same religion, different tribe. Sephardic cuisine also makes liberal use of cumin, cinnamon, saffron, dates, lentils, eggplant, and tomatoes. These are the flavors I understand and hunger for, hungered for before I even knew what they were. I was in the angstiest throes of my teens (my mother can tell you stories) when I learned you could cook this way and still be Jewish. Suddenly, I belonged somewhere. Suddenly, everything blossomed and made sense.

Okay, not everything. But I'm still drawn to the food of these countries. I must have the warming scent of cumin, the sweetness of cinnamon, in my kitchen; I must have these flavors in my mouth. Making recipes with origins dating back centuries, cooking food our forebears made in their kitchens, makes my heart replete.

I feel a kinship to those who came before, feel their presence with me as I make the food they made. They settle in, draping the folds of their robes around them just so, and watch me prepare the barley, chop the mint.

Because it is my fantasy, they are wise and warm and kind, and not hampered by the fact we don't speak the same language. They offer little suggestions. Add more lemon juice. Chop the mint a little finer. And because human nature has not changed so much over the centuries, they throw in a little critique or two. Who taught you to hold a knife that way? And why are your fingernails blue? If they're a little weirded out by my kitchen gear and getup, they recognize the barley salad, welcome and eat it.

I may be a little dodgy on the formal religion, but I kind of get into biblical, into old-school, into authenticity. This is, perhaps, what prompted me to make homemade matzo at Passover.

Matzo, or unleavened bread, is a thin, dry cracker sometimes known as the bread of faith, so you can understand how I'd be all over it. More often, though, it is called the bread of affliction. Call it what you will, there's only so much you can do with it. But what if you bake your own? It's a vital connection to our Jewish ancestors, has to taste better than your basic boxed matzo, and made with only flour, water, salt, and sometimes a little oil, it's pretty straightforward. It couldn't be too time-consuming — the Jews fleeing Egypt thousands of years ago had to bake the original matzo double-quick before blowing town. How hard could it be?

Famous last words.

To start with, there's the eighteen-minute rule. According to rabbinical law, there can be no chance for the dough to ferment and rise during baking. Therefore, from the time the flour hits the water to the time you take it out of the oven, making matzo must take less time than it takes to walk a Roman mile — clocked at eighteen minutes.

I measured out my flour and readied my rolling pin. At the bell, I set off in a matzo-making mania and wound up with a crispy, toasty matzo — flat and oblong and sometimes a little oddly shaped. It did not taste like cardboard. Olive oil made it delicious, and with a food processor (so much for old-school), it's doable in seventeen and a half minutes. Eureka, it's possible.

It is not, however, Passover worthy. My kitchen is clean, but it is not kosherized, which involves steaming or superheating all surfaces and utensils and having a rabbi bless the kitchen. I hadn't done any of that. I had a feeling I'd innocently committed a few other matzo misdemeanors, as well.

For instance, there's the flour issue. I used unbleached, all-purpose wheat flour. Wheat, along with barley, spelt, rye, and oats, has a gift for leavening. This quality makes it desirable for baking the rest of the year but is off-limits at Passover.

Millet, though, isn't on the ix-nay list. Most people know it only as birdseed, but this whole grain was big in Egypt centuries ago; and some food historians believe ground millet was used for that first-ever batch of matzo. Maybe I'd get by with a technicality if I made matzo with millet flour.

It mixed into a creamy batter and baked into a beautiful golden cracker, all within the limited time. But to taste, it was truly the bread of affliction. Millet matzo is brittle and sour.

Quinoa flour matzo? Doesn't seem like anything the ancient Jews had in mind (or at hand). I asked around and was met with your classic Yiddish shrug. Finally, I turned to a rabbi. Not just any rabbi, a Lubavitcher rabbi, as old-school as you can get.

"So, rabbi," I said. "How do I do it?"

The rabbi stroked his beard and sighed. "This I cannot advise."

It's not a flour issue. After all, commercial Passover matzo is made with wheat flour. What you need is a high-speed matzo-baking team and a commercial oven. At home by yourself, you can't keep turning out matzo fast enough or keep your oven hot enough.

"Make your own matzo? What do you need with that headache?" the rabbi said.

To re-create the ancestral experience, I explained. Tradition, connection, authenticity, faith, all that stuff.

"Keep the faith, buy the matzo," the rabbi said.

Did I listen?

DIY Matzo

I have experimented with many different kinds of flour (and abandoned millet flour altogether), and my personal best matzo uses both all-purpose and whole wheat flour. This combination wins for the dough that's easiest to handle and the matzo most worth eating. The recipe has its origins with the Jews who fled Egypt, but also with the estimable How to Cook Everything *author, Mark Bittman, who makes a stylish DIY matzo of his own.*

Matzo keeps in an airtight container for a day or two but tastes best right out of the oven.

Makes 1 dozen matzo, rustic and biblical in appearance and not at all bad to eat

¾ cup water
3 tablespoons olive oil
1 cup unbleached all-purpose flour
1 cup whole wheat flour
Sea salt for sprinkling

Preheat the oven to 500°F. Set out two baking sheets and have them ready for quick rollout-to-oven turnaround.

In a small bowl, whisk together the water and oil until it emulsifies, about 1 minute. Put the flours into a blender or food processor. With the motor running, slowly pour in the water-and-oil mixture. Blitz the mixture until a ball of smooth, not sticky, dough forms, about 1 minute.

Divide the dough into a dozen pieces. On a floured surface, roll out one piece of dough into a thin-as-possible round (or often in my case, a lopsided ovoid) about 8 inches across. Do not even think of rolling out more than one piece of matzo dough at a time — it won't work. Place gently on an ungreased baking sheet and sprinkle with salt. Prick the dough all over with a fork to prevent bubbles — a sign of leavening.

Repeat with the remaining pieces of dough.

Bake the matzo for 4 minutes on one side, or until golden brown and pebbled with brown, then gently flip, baking 4 minutes more.

Set on racks to cool.

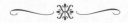

MY HEART IS FUL

Call it matzo, call it flatbread; it has applications well beyond Passover. My answer to the Arab-Israeli conflict is to use the matzo as an edible scoop for ful.

Someone needs to come up with a better name. But ful, or fava beans, the national dish of Egypt, dates back centuries, and you don't want to mess with anyone's beloved tradition. Even when it has an off-putting name that is sometimes, lamentably, spelled f-o-u-l.

Spell it any way you like, ful is not upmarket. It's "everyman's breakfast, the shopkeeper's lunch, and the poor man's dinner," as the Arabic saying goes, and a bowl of ful is a welcome sight at any time of the day.

This is not to say it is pretty. Alas, it is a bowl of brown, although sometimes you can add a few quick-cooking red lentils for color. But the beans are slow cooked until they yield, turning them kind and velvety in the mouth. Ful is toasty, nutty, primal, reminding us yet again that gentle heat and time work in concert to transform the humblest food into something to stir the soul.

Sometimes the beans are mashed until fluffy, then pretty much left alone, to enjoy as a dip or as one of the cooked vegetable salads of the Middle East. Sometimes ful is cooked with tomatoes, lemon, garlic, and cumin, the wonderful warming spice of Egypt, in which case it is called ful mudammas.

You can top ful with any number of garnishes, from tahini to chopped tomatoes and onions, or just with a drizzle of gutsy, green olive oil and a sprinkle of salt, but it is not to be tarted up. You'd be missing the point. This is the people's food. Egypt's national dish is not lamb, but a legume. A pot of ful feeds many and supplies a lot of protein and fiber for just a few piastres.

If there is anything unsatisfying about favas, it is this — the beans have a tough outer carapace that needs to be peeled before eating. To make matters worse, some people have an extreme allergic reaction to fava skins, called favism, not to be confused with fauvism, the French avant-garde art movement of a century ago. Very few people have been allergic to Matisse.

Available in Middle Eastern markets and many natural food stores, dried favas come in small, medium, and large, but the Egyptians wisely use only the small, tender ones for making ful. I have gone with a larger, lima-size fava, thinking fewer beans per pound would save me peeling time. I was sorely misguided. The bigger the bean, the tougher the skin and the greater the peeling effort. Small favas, which the Egyptians call ful hammam, or bath beans, are not only quicker to cook but easier to peel.

Whatever size favas you use, your best bet is to parboil the beans, peel them, then finish cooking until the beans are tender. I am sorry to tell you this can take as long as twelve hours. The final cooking, however, takes only minutes.

Ful is also sold in cans, if you want to spare yourself some time and labor, but you'll be cheating yourself out of the full ful experience. Peeling a pound of favas is a worthy endeavor, especially if you enlist others to help you.

In fact, peeling favas together in the same room is the ideal way to solve the Arab-Israeli conflict, marital conflict, any conflict. It keeps everyone's hands busy but leaves you free to converse, argue, understand, and ultimately feed each other. You may get frustrated with the process, but if you want to eat, you have to peel. Should diplomatic channels fail, the worst thing you can do is pelt each other with cooked beans.

I would much rather send generals into the kitchen to peel favas than send them into battle with guns, bombs, and brave, selfless troops. My new slogan — make ful, not war.

Peeling, when it comes to favas, is all about reaching the point of tenderness. Peeling, in all cases, is a revelation of self. And then we can sit down and eat together.

Ful Mudammas

Traditionally, each simple bowl of beans is topped with a goodly drizzle of olive oil, but to eat like an Egyptian, allow each person to salt his own ful.

This recipe doubles easily and can be served with homemade matzo or any flatbread that pleases you.

Serves 4

3 cups small fava beans cooked as per master plan (see
   page 16), or for an easier way, two 15-ounce cans ful,
   rinsed
4 cloves garlic, chopped
½ cup red lentils

1½ cups Stone Soup (see page 84) or other vegetable broth,
  water, or reserved fava bean cooking liquid
2 teaspoons ground cumin
2 tomatoes, chopped, or one 15-ounce can diced tomatoes,
  drained
Juice of 1 lemon
½ cup chopped fresh flat-leaf parsley
Olive oil for garnish (optional)
Tahini for garnish (optional)
Chopped fresh flat-leaf parsley and chopped tomatoes for
  garnish (optional)
Chopped scallions for garnish (optional)

In a medium saucepan, heat the cooked fava beans over medium-high heat. Add the garlic, lentils, broth, cumin, and tomatoes. Reduce the heat to medium and simmer, stirring occasionally, until everything starts to come together and the red lentils become tender, about 12 minutes.

Stir and smoosh until you get the consistency you like. Some people like their ful totally creamy, others more on the beany side. Stir in the lemon juice and ½ cup parsley. (The ful can be stored in an airtight container in the refrigerator up to 1 week; bring to room temperature just before serving.)

Top with your choice of garnishes, such as olive oil, tahini, parsley, tomatoes, and scallions.

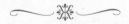

GENTLE NUDGE *the* FOURTH:
REDEFINING COMFORT

You look like you could be a chocolate person, but a little more interesting. Yeah? So let's say your comfort food of choice is turbofudge ice cream with salted toffee chunks. The coldness, the sweetness, the pop of saltiness, the clever interplay between the crunch of toffee and the coat-your-throat creaminess of the ice cream makes your eyes glaze with pleasure.

Or perhaps you're more of a mac-and-cheese sort. Creamy gets you off, too, but it has to be savory — salty and fatty, with a warm sauce of cheese (or what passes for it) robing noodles that ain't seen al dente in a while.

In both cases, these foods are so easy to eat, you barely have to chew. And you barely have to think, not if the manufacturers have done their job right. That salty/fatty/sweet flavor combination you love? Food companies love it, too, because it spikes your blood-sugar level and lights up all the pleasure receptors in your brain. This pretty light show comes with not-so-pretty consequences. It turns consumers into eating machines who don't question what the food is doing to them or to the environment. It turns us into junkies. Junkies are not good decision makers. Or rather, they're good at deciding all they want is more junk.

Within half an hour of eating your favorite indulgence, you hit comedown. Your blood sugar falls, along with your energy — and perhaps your self-image because you realize, congratulations, you've just loaded up on saturated fats, processed sugar, extra salt, and empty calories, plus a few chemical compounds you can't pronounce, let alone comprehend. Where's the comfort in that?

How food makes you feel is as important as how it tastes. Where it gets confusing is the emotional component — the "I want, I want, I want"s — having positive associations with food that promises comfort but lies to you. I hate liars.

How do you define comfort food? For me, it's something nourishing and pleasurable, energizing when I'm feeling good, propping me up when I'm needing support. That means something green and leafy; but serve a bowl of spinach to someone who's being visited by the Crap Fairy, and in most cases, you will not be greeted warmly, despite all your good intentions.

While I usually want something spicy or crunchy like a twenty-ingredient curry, in times when I'm in need of comfort, I want something simple to make and simple to eat, gentle in spicing, soft in texture, tender, because I want to be treated tenderly.

I want the pleasure of something sweet but would like to reduce the degree to which we are enslaved by processed sugar and flour, your basic white devils. Being vegan, I am also at odds with dairy and eggs. I ask a lot.

The vegan factor complicates everything. Many vegan baked goods are — and I don't want to alienate my own here — heavy. Or wet. Or both. My definitive zucchini bread recipe came about the way all my culinary successes do — off book, intuitively, in a kitchen fever. It is flavorful, flaxen, light, lemony, tender, and vegan, with eye-catching green zucchini flecks.

Zucchini bread multitasks, combining the sweet innocence of nursery food, the virtue of vegetables, and enough of a woo-hoo fun factor to make it all worthwhile.

Zucchini Bread

Enjoy with a cup of tea. Enjoy with someone you love. This can be yourself. Focus on the tea's gentle, floral notes, the bread's light and lemony sweetness. One small zucchini will do the trick. You'll have the benefit of its goodness but barely know it's there at work. Breathe. Feel at peace with the season, at peace with yourself. I'm not saying you have to sing "Kumbaya" or anything, but hey, if the spirit moves you.

¼ cup canola or coconut oil, plus more for oiling the pan
1 small zucchini, grated
2 tablespoons ground flaxseeds (also known as flax meal)
Zest and juice of 1 lemon
1½ cups spelt flour
1 tablespoon ground cinnamon
1 teaspoon baking soda
1 teaspoon aluminum-free baking powder
⅓ cup brown sugar
½ cup unsweetened soy milk
3 tablespoons agave nectar or maple syrup

Preheat the oven to 350°F. Lightly oil a 9-x-5-inch loaf pan.

In a small bowl, stir together the zucchini, flaxseeds, and lemon zest.

In a large bowl, sift together the spelt flour, cinnamon, baking soda, baking powder, and brown sugar.

Add the zucchini mixture to the flour mixture and toss, keeping things light — good advice for life in general.

In another small bowl, combine the soy milk and lemon juice. It will curdle; don't fret. Stir in the ¼ cup oil and agave nectar.

Gently stir the wet ingredients into the zucchini-flour mixture, until just combined.

Pour into the prepared loaf pan. Bake for 45 minutes, or until bread is golden and puffed, and a tester inserted in the center comes away crumb-free and clean. You can also give it a gentle poke with a finger; it should spring back when baked through.

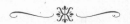

MOTHER'S DAY *for* DUMMIES ·

Spring is the season for regeneration, but it is also the season for she who generates. In April, we honor Mother Earth on Earth Day, then come May, we honor our own respective mothers on Mother's Day. Gotta love 'em both because without the planet and without your mom, you wouldn't be here.

Every year on Earth Day, we suddenly remember, oh, right, the earth is our home, where we've been getting room and board. For free. We feel guilty, so we throw parties, and they're fabulous; but the presents are even better, with people launching new green initiatives every year. The thing is, whether your community starts a composting program or you make your own pledge to buy and eat local produce at least twice a week, the earth gets it. She doesn't nag and say why haven't you called. She's the world's greatest mom. You don't need to take her out for brunch, just show some appreciation, make a little effort.

Jesus, it is said, made wine from water and fashioned loaves and fishes from thin air. The rest of us usually acquire foodstuffs by more conventional means. But for Earth Day, miracles are on the menu. You can help heal the planet, save money, and get a head start on dinner all in one go. I'll even throw in a story.

One brisk spring morning, a stranger appears in a village (one of your classic plotlines, by the way). The stranger's looking a little worse for wear and the village not much better. There's been war, famine, poverty; in fact, all the horsemen of the apocalypse have ridden through, and it's made the townsfolk a little less than friendly. They suggest the man move along.

"Right away," he says, "but I'd like to stop for something to eat first."

"Good luck," they say. "You won't be finding any food here."

He smiles. "No problem. Got everything I need right here. I'm in the mood for stone soup." He builds a small fire, fills a beat-up pot with water, and drops in what he says is his magic soup stone.

Magic and soup — these are both appealing things to those suffering hardship, and within minutes, the whole ragtag village has assembled to watch. The man stirs the pot and smiles. "Love a good stone soup," he says. "But, you know, what really makes it special is a bit of cabbage."

"Is that right?" One of the villagers produced a sorry-looking head of it.

"Great," the stranger says. He chops up the cabbage and adds it to the pot. "Thanks for helping me. You'll have some soup with me when it's ready, won't you?"

The villager is thrilled, also hungry.

Another villager asks what else goes into stone soup.

"Carrots are lovely, perhaps an onion, a potato, and I always like to add some greens — just like the kind growing around here."

Pretty soon the whole village has ponied up a vegetable or two to be chopped up and added to the pot with the magic soup stone. It all comes together to be a rich, life-sustaining soup the entire village can enjoy.

The moral is, we are capable of change, but only by working together. One twirly compact fluorescent bulb will not change the world. But if we all use them, they can help, and create a glow besides. So here is a stone soup for a Mother's Day for the mother of all.

Earth Day Special: Stone Soup (No Rocks Required), a.k.a. Vegetable Broth

Rather than tossing scraps and the odd bits of vegetables left over from cooking, throw them all in a bag — like a gallon-size plastic one. Extra points if you use environmentally friendly reusable bags, available at most natural food stores.

Throw the bag in the freezer. Add scraps to the bag every time you chop fresh herbs, peel an onion, or tear up greens for a salad. Carrot, tomato, and potato peels, green bean tops and tails, stemmy bits of parsley and cilantro, cabbage cores, woody broccoli stems — everything goes in the bag. When it's full and you've got an hour or so, it's broth-making time.

Dump the veggie bits into a soup pot — two gallons or larger. Add four cups of water, a cup or two more if you've reached vegetable scrap mother lode. Put the lid on the pot, set the burner on high, and let the water come to a boil. Turn off the heat, leave the pot in place for half an hour (or longer), and you are done.

Meanwhile, the veggie bits and hot water will coalesce, producing gorgeous vegetable broth. Known as passive cooking, it may look like you're doing nothing, but you're making broth and saving energy, both yours and the electricity or gas necessary to heat the soup. Keeping the lid on means the heat doesn't escape and does the work for you.

Let the mixture cool, then strain the broth through a sieve or colander into a waiting pot. Vegetable broth can be frozen until you're ready to use it. Compost cooked and cooled scraps.

Taste varies based on whatever goes into the broth. However, it's always better than the purchased stuff. There's no salt unless/until you add it. And you never have to lay out another penny for prepared vegetable broth again.

It's not a recipe to serve to guests, but you'll make it a lot, I hope. Use it instead of water to cook whole grains — vegetable broth infuses them with both nutrients and flavor. Use it as the base for soups and stews, and as the base for a home-cooked Mother's Day celebration.

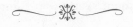

Along with Valentine's Day and New Year's Eve, Mother's Day is a holiday to be spent with those you love, at home — your home, your friend's home, your relative's home, anyone's home. Just don't go out to a restaurant.

These holidays, where we are called upon to be our truest, most authentic and adorable selves, turn restaurants, even those where the rest of the year they live to serve, into crazed money-making gouge machines.

Okay, so perhaps I have issues, especially with brunch buffets. I'm still recovering from the trauma of my first, which should have been a spectacular fairy tale of a feast.

I must have been eight when my parents took me to San Francisco. I fell in love with the sea lions off Fisherman's Wharf. My mother fell in love with the idea of having brunch at the Fairmont. And so we went. We were greeted, seated at a table with thick white linens, then directed to the food.

Well, you couldn't miss it, could you? There were tiers of it. Sausages sweating red under heat lamps, whole fish sculpted to look as though leaping from their platters. There were baskets upon baskets of pastries; bakeries had been raided of their breads. Bowls heaped with mayonnaise-begooped salads flanked a tower of pancakes dripping with meringue.

I wonder how it would look to me now. I only know that as a kid, I found it terrifying.

I went through the buffet line, holding my empty plate in front of me with both hands.

My parents offered me food from this platter, that bowl, gave the tooth-baring smiles that signal parental encouragement.

"You can have whatever you want," they said.

What I wanted was to go home, back to Miami, back to our house, where things made sense and things had scale. I sensed

going home was not an option right then, nor would it go down
well if I so much as proposed it.

I proceeded to the end of the line. I went back. I might have
walked around for a very long time. By the time I returned to the
platter of meringue-topped pancakes — why would you *do* that
to a pancake? — they had been picked over, leaving an oozing
puddle of oneness; the leaping fishes' bones were exposed. And
sharp. The mayonnaisey things had only grown whiter and wetter.

I brought my plate back to my smiling parents (who, for all I
know, had already gone back for seconds), smoothed the napkin
over my lap like a big girl, and was about to eat the feast of my
choosing, when a man, another brunch patron, bent over me and
said, "Is that all you're going to eat, little girl? You know, your
father has spent a lot of money to bring you here."

I then looked from the small cluster of green grapes and the
single red-dyed crabapple on my plate to the man. His voice was
kind, though firm, his sport jacket plaid and loud. I burst into
tears.

I was a kid. I didn't understand the ways of food justice; I just
knew there was no way we could eat all this food. How hungry
could any of us be? Worse, no one truly hungry and in need was
going to get any of it, either. A lose-lose situation.

My father drew himself up and said, "My daughter can eat
whatever she wants."

Score one for dad. It was as though he'd lifted me onto his
shoulders.

But who was going to stand up for everyone else?

I plucked a green grape from its cluster, sucking it in with
an audible pop. But it couldn't eclipse a new hatred of brunch, a
horror of waste, and a wariness of men in plaid sport coats. I have
outgrown none of them.

Oh, there's some tasteful-enough sport coats out there, and some guys can carry the look; but with the waste thing, there's no question — food is not necessarily a case where more is better, especially when half gets tossed.

The question is, what makes a feast? The answer for my mother and aunt, children of Depression parents, is plenty. They both suffer nightmares of running out of food. This has never, ever happened, and yet that fear is still there. They compensate by serving if not overabundance, then let us say generous portions, and Benjamin and I always leave with bags of leftovers.

The ancient Romans ate until they were ill, politely excused themselves to hurl, then returned to the table. An interesting over-the-top attitude, but they didn't last as a civilization. Some Japanese practice *hara hachi bu*, eating until you're 80 percent full. This may seem like it'd do you in, too. But in Japan, food is art. It's plated to delight the eye. Your stomach gets its fill, but so do your senses.

I lack the patience — and knife skills — to carve a carrot into a rose but don't mind spending time in the kitchen preparing food or at the table enjoying it. Time is a crucial ingredient to creating a feast. It may be no more than a pot of jasmine tea shared with a friend. It's less about the food you eat than the spirit and attention you bring to it. Taking time to eat can seem like a luxury, but the alternative isn't pretty.

Our first two years of married life, Benjamin and I lived in Tokyo. Lunchtime in the business district was observed with a sort of brief, frantic horror. Tokyo businessmen slurped down their soba in seconds. They flipped their ties aside, raised bowls to their mouths, and emptied the broth — still steaming — and the tangle of noodles in one rapid go. Delight the eye it did not. It probably didn't do much for their digestion, either.

You don't want to look like that. And you don't want to feel like that. Slowing down rather than speed-eating invites you to become aware of the physical sensation of eating, one of life's great unsung pleasures. So why rush it? Indulge in feeling the silky soba noodles slip around in your mouth, contrast that with the thin, crisp disks of carrot, the meaty chew of shiitakes. Feel the heat of the broth, taste the brininess from the soy, the gentle bite from the ginger, the gauziest overlay of fermentation from the miso.

Eating slowly also makes you recognize that moment of fullness, poised between *hara hachi bu* and ancient Roman excess. That is the beautiful moment of *enough*, when you feel that happy *ahh* in the belly and the soul and need nothing more. The "more, more, more" urge will set in soon enough. For now, try to enjoy the moment. Breathe. It helps.

The technical word is *satiety*, or fullness, and it sounds to me very like the Arabic benediction said at the beginning or end of a meal — *sahtayn*, wishing two healths to you. You deserve at least two healths. So does your mother. So does Mother Earth. So make Mother's Day meaningful, mindful, a day of celebration, not waste. A simple (meatless) meal prepared with a whole heart beats a more-than-you-can-eat and more-than-you-can-afford buffet.

Show Mom the love. Show her the lunch. Make it yourself.

Kamut for Mother Earth

Here's a whole grain dish I created that earned the seal of approval from my mother and aunt. It's made with Kamut, or khorasan wheat. It's ancient whole grain, so ancient it's believed to have originated in the Fertile Crescent, and takes its name from a hieroglyph. It's got all its ancient goodness intact and even wheat-sensitive folks seem able to enjoy it. There's much to enjoy — a rich, nutty taste and terrific chew. You've been meaning to eat more whole grains anyway. It can be made a day or two ahead, so it makes things easy for you. And it's organic, so it makes Mother Earth happy, too.

Kamut for Mother Earth

Kamut needs to be soaked in water overnight and requires slow cooking. Don't fuss about it too much, just factor in a little time.

Serves 4 to 6, doubles like a dream

3 cups Stone Soup (see page 84) or other vegetable broth

1 cup Kamut (also known as khorasan wheat)

1 clove garlic

2 bay leaves

4 to 5 carrots, coarsely chopped

2 onions, coarsely chopped

2 tablespoons olive oil

2 tablespoons Dijon mustard, plus more as needed

Juice of 2 lemons, plus more as needed

1 bunch Swiss chard or a good handful fresh spinach or
  arugula leaves, chopped

1 bunch fresh flat-leaf parsley, chopped

1 tablespoon chopped fresh tarragon (if you're a big dill
  fan, swap it for tarragon)

Sea salt and freshly ground pepper

In a large pot, bring the broth to a boil. Meanwhile, pour the Kamut into a sieve and rinse with cold water. When the broth boils, add the rinsed Kamut, the garlic, and bay leaves. Cover, reduce the heat to low, and simmer for 1½ hours. I know, it's a long time, but the Kamut keeps its own company. When the grains have plumped up enormously and are tender and chewy, the Kamut is ready.

Meanwhile, you can do other things while the Kamut cooks. For instance, you can preheat the oven to 350°F.

Spread the carrots and onions on a large rimmed baking sheet. Drizzle with 1 tablespoon of the olive oil. Roast until fragrant, slightly darkened, and just tender, about 30 minutes, giving the vegetables an occasional flip or stir so they roast evenly.

In a small bowl, whisk together the 2 tablespoons Dijon mustard, the remaining 1 tablespoon olive oil, and the juice of 2 lemons.

Transfer the cooked Kamut to a large bowl. Add the chard, herbs, and roasted vegetables along with their liquids. Pour the mustard-and-lemon dressing over all and mix again.

Season with salt and pepper. Taste and zing up with a little more mustard or lemon juice, if desired.

Serve at room temperature or hot. The Kamut for Mother Earth can be stored in an airtight container in the refrigerator for several days; reheat just before serving. To reheat, bake covered at 350°F for about 30 minutes, stirring occasionally.

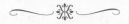

GENTLE NUDGE *the* FIFTH: GO OLD-SCHOOL

Kamut, farro, spelt, quinoa, millet, barley, amaranth — this isn't a magical incantation. Or maybe it is. The words are names for ancient grains, whole grains that have been around for centuries. For centuries, whole was how we ate grain, too. Then we discovered milling.

Milling, or grinding, grain removed the husk. It rendered the grain softer, easier to chew, easier to digest. Milling was originally done by hand, a difficult job that made processed grain expensive. It became the food of the privileged, a status symbol — refined grain for refined people.

Over the centuries, it became more affordable, more available, and still we processed. It's only been within the past half century that we've realized just how nutritionally neutered refined grain is. Whole grain has its kernel and bran intact, and that's where the hard-core nutrients are. That's where the fiber, the fun-for-the-mouth chew, and the nutty, earthy flavor are, too.

We are a nation absorbed by youth, radiant health, and beauty. And yet the majority of us are fat, sick, and not hot. This was nothing we flash-mobbed. It's the result of what we eat. And it's not entirely our fault. Many of us have been raised on processed, refined white flour, white rice, white bread. They're fluffy, cheap, bland, and some nutritionists believe they're the reason so many people are suffering from wheat intolerance. What's for sure, though, is refined grains contribute to the triple threat of diabetes, heart disease, and cancer. Not too yum.

We're so taken with foods that claim to be natural and healthful on the label, we overlook foods that really are. Give ancient grains a try. They're your age-old sources for great energy, nourishment, flavor, and satiety (that's that happy, full-belly feeling). Even without a label that says so. Rediscover ancient grains. Eat them in all their robust, unrefined glory.

Farrotto with Greens, Pine Nuts, and Currants

Traditional risotto gets its luscious, chewy, creamy texture from short-grain arborio rice and constant stirring. This dish gives you the same terrific result with less effort and whole grain goodness, too. Call it far-rotto, call it Fred, this is a cheaty version of risotto made with farro.

To soak or not to soak, that is the question. Many chefs go straight ahead and cook the farro without soaking. I soak it overnight, and it comes out tremendously creamy and cooks up quickly. Try it both ways.

Serves 6

2 cups farro
¼ cup pine nuts
4 teaspoons olive oil
3 cloves garlic, minced
1 dried red pepper, crumbled, or a couple of good pinches
    of red pepper flakes
1 bunch Swiss chard, spinach, kale, or other hearty winter
    greens, chopped into bite-size pieces
5 cups Stone Soup (see page 84) or other vegetable broth or
    water
¼ cup currants
Sea salt and freshly ground pepper

Pour the farro into a sieve, rinse with cold water, and drain. In a large bowl, soak the farro in enough cold water to cover overnight (or not — your call).

Preheat the oven to 350°F.

Pour the pine nuts in a shallow ovenproof pan and toast until they just turn golden, about 6 minutes. They can go from golden to black in a matter of minutes, so watch the time carefully and zip them out of the oven as soon as they're ready. Transfer the pine nuts to a small bowl to cool.

In a stockpot, heat the olive oil over medium-high heat. Add the garlic and red pepper. Cook, stirring occasionally, until the garlic and red pepper sizzle and are fragrant, a few minutes. Add the chard, a handful at a time, and cook until it just wilts, 4 to 5 minutes. Transfer the chard to another large bowl.

No need to clean out the stockpot. Drain the farro and pour into the pot. Heat over medium-high heat. Stir until the farro toasts and gets a little luster from the residual oil, about 2 minutes.

Add the vegetable broth, stir, and bring to a boil.

Cover, reduce the heat to low, and simmer until most of the liquid is absorbed, about 30 minutes. (The farro will continue to soak up liquid as it cools.) The farro will be thick and creamy with a risotto-esque consistency.

Stir in the chard and the currants. The currants, which start out tiny and wrinkly, will plump up from the heat.

Season with salt and freshly ground pepper. Gently stir the pine nuts into the farro, reserving 1 tablespoon for garnish.

To serve, mound into a serving bowl or spoon onto individual plates. Sprinkle the last of the pine nuts on top.

The farrotto can be stored in an airtight container in the refrigerator for several days; reheat just before serving.

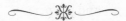

the GLOBAL STEW

As a fledgling existentialist in my tweens, I coined the Existential Stew Theory, which posits you are a carrot. Or an artichoke. Or a mushroom. Or a sprig of basil. You are significant, with your own character, your own unique flavor and qualities. You are whole and independent. Yet you are a necessary ingredient in an elaborate stew. Take away any one ingredient, and the dish suffers. But when you hang out with your fellow ingredients, you enhance each other, you bring out the best in each other. Together, we become even better than what we are individually. And isn't that the point of being human, to bump up against other humans and help each other out?

Not bad as a theory — it's reality where things get complicated. I would pay good money to avoid bumping up against some people. They do not bring out the best in me; they send my shoulders up around my ears and make me hiss like a cornered possum.

Apparently, other people feel the same way. About *me*. How can this be possible? But how else to explain the fence our next-door neighbors put up around their house? It is eight feet high, with wooden planks standing side by side, admitting no light in between. It totally encloses their home from view. It's a box around their house. What's next? A moat?

They call it a fence; I call it a corral. It might look more fitting out in the country. But we are not out in the country; we are smack dab in the middle of a city block, and their fence comes right up against the property line of our tiny lot. It casts unfortunate shadows in my backyard where my arugula would otherwise flourish. It's an affront to the eye. And it's such a snub. Perhaps the fence makes them feel safe. From what? From me? Obviously, my neighbors are deeply disturbed. Also misguided. Because if they think they can just shut me out, they've got another think coming.

There are also people you might prefer not to bump up against. But bump we do, and there's no fence big enough to keep us all apart. There are seven billion of us at the table now, and we're facing a case of too many mouths and not enough food. The world grows enough grain so every one of us seven billion can have two pounds of it per day, plus all the produce you can eat (and you should eat more than you do — just saying). Alas, a third or more of that grain goes to feeding livestock, while one out of every six of us goes hungry. With not enough for us all, the political, religious, economic, and cultural differences between us can appear large. And ugly. Fear and hatred make us not so pretty, either.

I don't mean you, of course. You are magnificent. But you are not the only flavor the world has to offer. We are all here to live. And it's not always easy.

I know what you're thinking — let's get all this eating and enlightenment stuff out of the way now, so I can get back to work, my family, my laundry, and maybe grab a coffee and a Pilates class. I'm so sorry. I wish it worked that way. If life and spirit and dinner could be reduced to a tweet, I'd be on it. But it takes time and patience to appreciate how it all connects. You have to relax into it. Patience and relaxation are nothing I'm good at, but I know you can't rush connection any more than you can hasten the slow-cooking magic that goes into a pot of stew.

Yes, stew. It turns out my twelve-year-old self had some wisdom. We are all together in the great global stew. We depend on each other. Not as directly as we did when our ancestors took in strangers, but just as much. Not loving each other madly doesn't change that. Putting up stupid-ass fences between us doesn't change that, either.

So I try to breathe and be my bigger, better self, to deal with our differences with some compassion, some humility. And some dinner.

Of course, what happens in a church or a mosque or a synagogue matters, but I'm more interested in the food we share when we come home. Almost every religion, every culture, has its own holiday soup or stew. It may contain a spice or seasoning that's not in your pantry — or comfort zone; but strip away the differences, and you have a pot of commonality, ingredients every culture knows. They're rich in tradition but easy on the belly, simple and sustaining.

Stews are cultural comfort food; they are the people's food. This is food that takes down the fences we build between us, that bridges our otherness. Good thing, too. We all gotta eat. In the synchronistic way life sometimes has when you play your cards right, I discovered gumbo z'herbes, New Orleans's amazing green gumbo, in the spring, when collards, chard, spinach, watercress, sorrel, parsley, tatsoi, kale, dandelion, mustard, and turnip greens all conspire to explode from my garden, community-supported agriculture (CSA) box, and farmers' market.

I can't tell the kale, "Not now, darling. Come back next week," or ask the collards to please shrink down from their elephant-ear size to something more manageable. Not only is it peak season for greens in my part of the world, but this überabundance happens at the right season as far as the Catholic Church is concerned.

Silly, heathen me, I'd been smitten with it because it tasted so good and made me feel so good. Who knew it could be penance grub? It turns out gumbo z'herbes is an Ash Wednesday tradition, complying with the Lenten abstinence from meat. Carnival, as Mardi Gras is also known, comes from the Latin *carne vale* — literally, "farewell, meat." Please note it does not mean "farewell, fun." Gumbo z'herbes is meatless, but it shows your mouth a good time. It takes the sting out of forty days of prayer and austerity. You can enjoy in good faith. Truly.

You can, as I did, pronounce it with a French accent, but in Louisiana, they looked at me as if I was crazy. There, they say "gumbo zav." And they created it, so who am I to argue? And I can't argue with any recipe that lets me use leafy and so-called lowly greens, spin them into culinary gold, and make room in my refrigerator, too. We're talking a lot of greens. Pounds of them, as many kinds as you like, as long as they're an odd number. This is believed to bring good fortune, and if not exactly sanctioned by the Catholic Church, it makes a good story. I think we're as hungry for narrative as we are for food. Or maybe that's just me.

If you prefer your meal without backstory and religious significance, gumbo z'herbes will still come through for you. It's crazy with calcium, iron, antioxidants, and whatnot. But you also get your RDA of a kind of nourishment even collards can't supply — the nourishment of the spirit. Fulfillment, joy, connection are built right in.

Here's another opportunity to use your vegetable broth. It's a time investment — you don't want to rush a roux. There's something leisurely, expansive, luxurious about making gumbo z'herbes, and you know, when you spend the time making food, you're well on your way to a feast. If you've got a food processor, you've got it made. Most of the work happens in the pot without your help, and the result is amazing. It's a labor of love with a big flavor payoff — just what you'd want to make for people you care about. Serve over cooked brown rice; keep your favorite hot sauce handy.

CSA Gumbo Z'herbes

Gumbo z'herbes is green gumbo — just what kind of green is up to you and what's fresh and available. I use what comes in my community supported agriculture box — escarole, collards, tatsoi, rainbow chard, and beet greens. Remember, use an odd number of greens for good luck.

Traditionally, gumbo z'herbes is ladled over white rice. I prefer brown rice, both for its nutty flavor and its greater, grainier nourishment. Either way, this gumbo makes a big, serious bowl of green.

Serves 8 to 10

5 big bunches greens (escarole, collards, tatsoi, chard, beet
  greens — whatever's green and fresh)
Table salt for the greens
⅓ cup plus 2 tablespoons olive oil
½ cup whole wheat flour
2 onions, coarsely chopped
6 cloves garlic
4 stalks celery plus their leaves, coarsely chopped
2 red bell peppers, coarsely chopped
6 cups Stone Soup (see page 84) or other vegetable broth
1 handful fresh thyme leaves
1 bay leaf
¼ teaspoon cayenne pepper
1 tablespoon apple cider vinegar
Sea salt and freshly ground pepper

Wash your greens really, really well. This is the most important step, as a mouthful of grit is not pleasing. The best way I've found to clean greens is to plop them down and rinse them thoroughly in your sink. Then pick them over. You can reserve the odd stemmy bits for broth. Shake in some table salt and rinse again. (The salt helps rid the greens of stubborn sand and such.) Give a final rinse and blot dry.

The old-school method for cooking gumbo greens is to blanch or boil them, but I prefer steaming, which keeps their color bright and their lovely nutrients intact. Steam greens in batches in a covered steamer or double boiler. Fill the bottom pot halfway with water. Bring to a boil over high heat. Place the greens in the steamer inset, or the top pot of a double boiler, the one with the holes at the bottom.

Cover and steam so the greens are just tender yet still vibrant and bright colored. Time varies for the different greens. Soft-leafed greens like spinach steam in 3 to 5 minutes. Sturdier greens like collards may take twice as long.

Place the greens in a colander with a pot beneath them to catch all the good veggie broth.

Meanwhile, make your roux. In a large soup pot, heat ⅓ cup of the olive oil over very low heat. Whisk in the flour and cook, whisking occasionally, for a really long time, maybe 45 minutes, or until the roux starts to give off a toasty scent and turns chocolaty in color.

Meanwhile, in a food processor, pulse the onions and garlic until they're finely chopped, not mushy, about a minute, tops. In a large skillet, heat the remaining 2 tablespoons olive oil over medium heat. Stir in the onion-garlic mixture.

One by one, finely chop the celery, bell peppers, and, finally, the greens, in the food processor, add to the skillet, and stir to combine. Once the vegetables start to soften and coalesce, in 5 to 7 minutes, give them a last stir, then reduce the heat to low. Cover, and cook for 20 minutes or so, stirring occasionally, until vegetables are welcoming and tender.

Your roux and vegetables are now ready to meet each other. Gently stir the vegetable mixture into the roux, until everything is well combined. Raise the heat to medium-high and add the vegetable broth plus any juices from the drained greens. Add the thyme, bay leaf, and cayenne. When the mixture starts to boil, cover, reduce the heat to medium-low, and cook, stirring occasionally, for 1 hour more, or until the gumbo darkens and thickens a little more. Oh, don't complain; be generous of spirit. Call a friend, check your e-mail, pour yourself a glass of wine, if it helps.

Splash in the vinegar and season with sea salt and pepper.

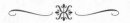

GENTLE NUDGE *the* SIXTH: SEASON *to* TASTE

You could call the way this riot of fresh greens coincides with Lent divine intervention, a great cosmic meant-to-be. Or you could call it seasonality. This term has gotten a lot of buzz in the past few years, which goes to show you how out of whack we are. Until the last century, seasonal eating was all we did. We would harvest the fruits and vegetables available to us when they were ripe and ready. Some we dried and stored for winter, but most we'd eat right then. This makes sense.

Then came refrigeration and air travel, and we could get fresh grapes in December. We could get everything all the time. And we still weren't happy. Because the grapes didn't much taste like grapes, as they were grown for sturdiness rather than for that low, slow building of tannic skin and sweet, juicy flesh, and hint of soil and rain that's inherently grapy. The grapes were picked under-ripe so they wouldn't be dead by the time they got to you, then they were flown or trucked in from another country.

International travel totally rags me out, so how can it not do the same to a grape?

Then there's the cost for out-of-season stuff. The earth has limited amounts of oil, limits we're bumping up against. Depleting our finite reserves for a bunch of grapes because the mood strikes is not, as your accountant will tell you, cost-efficient.

The problem is, we've gotten out of sync with the rhythms of the earth. Our go-go society makes us feel guilty for being other than 24/7, when really, lovey, no one is 24/7. Or if so, it's because whoever it is has staff. Even the planet doesn't do 24/7. Twenty-four/seven is a lie — there, I've said it.

But do we listen? Not from the looks of things. Eating out of season is like living in a foreign country without understanding the language. You might be able to get by with frantic gestures and shouting, but you miss the nuance, all the lovely ways of this place. You miss what the earth is trying to tell you. It's saying, pay attention. Live in the moment. Gather ye rosebuds — and broccoli buds and nasturtium buds — while ye may, because they won't be here tomorrow. Or if they're still around, they'll have lost their luster.

Luster is the best reason to eat what's ripe now. Think of fresh popcorn versus stale; flat champagne versus a bottle that bubbles and sparkles. Food tastes best when it's fresh. Seasonal eating is nature's way of directing you to food at its most vibrant, when it's crazy-mad with chi (Chinese for "life force"). It connects you to the earth and its seasons and throws a little meaning in, if you're looking for it. Mostly, though, it's about having a good time, about adding a little more luster to your life.

Roasted Beet Salad with Chili-Lime Vinaigrette

Beets, mangoes, and jicama (also known as Mexican turnip) are Mexican crops, and they feature in spring and summer salads like this one, sparked with a chili-lime vinaigrette. It's suitable for Cinco de Mayo and pretty enough for Mother's Day.

Serves 4 to 6

2 good-size beets (save greens for soup or for sautéing —
    you know how I feel about waste)
Juice of 2 limes
1 tablespoon balsamic vinegar or apple cider vinegar
2 teaspoons agave nectar or honey

3 tablespoons olive oil

1 teaspoon Dijon mustard

1 teaspoon ground cumin

½ teaspoon chili powder

3 to 4 bunches fresh baby greens (arugula, butter lettuce,
watercress, or spinach)

½ jicama (also known as Mexican turnip), peeled and
diced, or 1 young white turnip, peeled and diced

1 orange, peeled and cut into bite-size pieces

1 mango, peeled and chopped (if available)

⅓ cup almonds or pecans, toasted and coarsely chopped

1 bunch fresh cilantro, chopped

Preheat the oven to 400°F.

Wash the beets, wrap them tightly in aluminum foil, and roast
for 1 hour. Remove from the oven and let cool. When the beets are
cool enough to handle, slip off the skins and chop into bite-size
pieces. (The chopped, roasted beets can be wrapped and stored in
the refrigerator for a day.)

In a small bowl, whisk together the lime juice, balsamic vinegar,
agave nectar, olive oil, mustard, cumin, and chili powder. You should
have about ⅓ cup of dressing, ample for this salad plus leftovers.

Arrange the greens on a platter or on individual plates. Top with
beets, jicama, orange, mango (if using), almonds, and cilantro.

Drizzle the dressing on top.

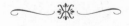

Chapter

3 *the* HARVEST

"Summer surprised us," writes T. S. Eliot. The phrase comes early in "The Waste Land," and it also surprises the reader, already so lost in the poem's rich layers as to be startled by these five simple syllables that come in the eighth line.

I still feel a kid's deep-hearted yearning in summer, an itch to be outside, to run till I flop down on the grass and pant like a dog. Summer in Miami is hot and wet-blanket humid. It is something you enter, like a sauna. The sun bleaches out the sky. Lawns crisp in the heat. So do the sunburned tourists, who stagger around, eyes vacant. Natives know enough to go inside and seek air-conditioning. On the upside, the riffraff have taken off, and we can get into our favorite restaurants without a reservation.

Summer surprises me, too. What surprises me is how quickly it goes. It's no sooner Memorial Day than it's Labor Day, and everyone's talking back-to-school this and that. Summer over, game over. I think of scripture, particularly the Old Testament, Jeremiah 8:20 — "The harvest is past, the summer is ended, and we are not saved." In other words, more than half the year is shot, and what have I got to show for it?

It was not always thus. Summers of childhood were open and endless. On Saturdays, my parents would rent a cabana, a fancy name for a bare, cement-floored roomette on the beach where they could unload their carload of stuff and me. I would run screaming into the water, the waves roughhousing me until my lips were salt numbed, my eyes stinging, and fingertips puckered. I could be counted on to drop my lunch in the sand, to run from my mother as she tried to slather me with sunscreen, and to howl as she rinsed off my coating of salt, sand, and sunscreen under the spray of the cold-water public shower.

On the Fourth of July, we'd stay into the evening. Separate families would gather and mingle, and a frenzied parade of dogs and children ran up and down the beach. We'd write our names in sparklers and set off fireworks, the big, lacy ones I loved and the boomy cannon-shot kind that got the boys revved and made me hide behind my parents. The fathers, of course, would grill. I don't know why Independence Day has become synonymous with incinerated meat. Something about the rockets' red glare? There would be hot dogs, with their upsetting name and more upsetting rubbery pink skin. Someone was always shuttling me away from my architecturally challenged sand castles to hand me a bun with a hot dog sporting a racing stripe of mustard. I liked ketchup. Dropping a peanut-butter-and-raspberry-jelly sandwich in the sand was tragic. Dropping a hot dog? No loss.

With the grilling came the attendant salads — potato salad and coleslaw. Potato salad was soft and white and bland, but it made sense. It was a salad made from potatoes. But what on earth was a *cole*? Whatever it was, it wasn't in the slaw, which was always, always, always shredded cabbage, carrots, and maybe some onion, bound by bottled mayonnaise and vinegar. Sometimes it featured celery seeds, a clear sign the cook was a bit of a rogue. Or a southerner.

The good part about getting older is sometimes you do attain some wisdom. Maybe not the secrets of the universe, but you learn that *cole* refers to vegetables of the mustard-green family, which includes cabbage (also kale, collards, broccoli, turnips, brussels sprouts, mustard greens, beloved to me all). You also learn you can slaw just about any fruit or vegetable and toss your edible confetti with things other than mayo.

This mayoless Moroccan carrot salad is one of my favorite summer dishes. It's seasonal, bright to the eye, bright with flavor, and absurdly easy to make. It needs just a little kitchen heat — a minute or two to toast the spices. And it stands up beautifully at a picnic or a day at the beach.

Moroccan Carrot Salad

Serves 6 to 8

1 pound carrots
1 tablespoon olive oil
1 teaspoon ground cumin
1 teaspoon ground paprika; sweet is traditional, smoked is
    edgy but quite nice
Generous pinch of cayenne pepper or, if you have it,
    Aleppo pepper
2 teaspoons agave nectar or honey
Juice of 1 or 2 lemons

½ teaspoon sea salt
1 bunch fresh flat-leaf parsley, coarsely chopped

Coarsely shred the carrots in a food processor or cut into ¼-inch matchsticks, your call. Dump into a good-size bowl and set aside.

In a small skillet, heat the oil, cumin, paprika, and cayenne over low heat, stirring now and again until spices darken and the whole thing turns fragrant, 2 to 3 minutes. Remove from the heat and let cool.

Pour the spiced oil over the carrots. Add the agave nectar, lemon juice, and sea salt, and stir until the carrots are evenly coated. (The carrot salad can be stored in an airtight container in the refrigerator for a day.)

Just before serving, gently stir in the parsley. Enjoy slightly chilled but not gelid.

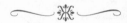

WHAT I LEARNED *in* SUMMER SCHOOL

Childhood summer stretched on even after the fireworks of the Fourth were over. Some of my friends went off to camp. I rather felt sorry for them. Summer unleashed in me a lightness, a license to *be*, rather than to do, to spend the day outside in the sun with dogs and books, and making my rounds to indulgent neighbors. Each day was simple, sweet and golden, like the single drop of nectar in an ixora blossom, and the whole world was my friend.

My parents do not even like the beach. They went to please me. And because they needed a diversion but couldn't afford a real vacation. My father sported sideburns in those days or in my memory, and the ocean was blue and high and fierce. It is so flat now. It is a softer blue, a calmer friend, its rowdy days all but forgotten. Or perhaps I'm the tame one now. Tamer and busier.

I do not heed the call of summer the way I did — too many things to get to. I have lost my girlhood gift for being here now. I am good at being at least fifteen minutes ahead and live in an anxious state of perpetual what-comes-next-ness. It keeps me in favor with editors because I never miss a deadline. It has kept me out of trouble the few times I've done commercial kitchen prep because I can keep up and not piss off the chef. I'm conscientious, reliable, but not patient. I am impatient with my own impatience, my own limitations.

I was ranting to a friend about this. She gave me one of her great Mona Lisa smiles and this advice: "Embrace your mess."

Are you kidding me? Oh, I know our strengths and our weaknesses are often two halves of the same. I have no trouble embracing *your* mess. Your mess is charming, your mess is just fine. It's my own that drives me forty kinds of crazy. On the list of character flaws: my out-of-the-box nervousness, my stupid tendency to want to be everybody's best friend, my resistance to doing things the easy way, my inability to cut myself some slack.

Change is possible. Radical character makeovers are tougher. The best I can hope for is to take a break from busting my butt, every now and again. Maybe just once a year. And summer is the time to do it, when I can learn from an excellent role model — the whole earth.

During the months when the earth and the sun are best buds, the planet itself takes a break. This is not winter dormancy. It's the promise of spring fulfilled; it's taking a holiday after a job well done. The warm temperature and warm light of summer say come out to play — the time is right, and the produce is ripe. We call fruits and vegetables "produce" because, well, the earth has produced them, sometimes with some help from us. So come. Eat. Wear sunscreen.

Here in my backyard, the collards keep going and growing, impervious to both cold and heat, their leaves as tough and big as elephant ears. The rest of my wee garden has yielded up its lot — heirloom tomatoes, odd shaped, sun warmed, and sweet; arugula, with its Victorian, scalloped leaves and punk pepper kick; long curls of red Russian kale; rainbow chard, with its clean, ozone taste, tender leaves, and neon-bright red-and-yellow stems.

Bees and zebra longwing butterflies zip in and out of our firebush, a lacy puff of red blossoms like the fireworks I love. Here is the open sky and benevolent sun. And here, minutes away, is the broad basin of the Atlantic, a phalanx of brown pelicans zooming just above the water, their wings fanned out, creating not so much as a ripple on the surface. A calm falls over me, and a smidge of space opens between my cervical vertebrae, usually tension fused into a state of oneness.

Embrace your mess — a lot of value in those three words.

Other useful three-word advice:

Be here now.

Breathe. It helps.

And there's what my father said to me right before he lowered my bridal veil and walked me down an absurd spiral staircase to waiting wedding guests and my groom — Don't fuck up.

I am constantly trying for all the above, to relearn what birds and insects know, what I once knew by instinct, knew from the inside — to live in the moment and be grateful for it.

Even Job, that miserable guy from the Bible, said:

> *But ask the animals, and they will teach you,*
> *or the birds of the air, and they will tell you;*
> *or speak to the earth, and it will teach you,*
> *or let the fish of the sea inform you.*

Which of all these does not know
that the hand of the Lord has done this?
In his hand is the life of every creature
and the breath of all mankind.

It is about letting go, surrendering, being vulnerable and open to possibility, expanding, inhabiting the moment rather than rushing through it on our way to somewhere else. Which is a great way to approach seasonal eating. (And you didn't think I could work this back around to food, did you?)

Barbecue is for other people. Summer for me is the sticky, sweet, in-your-face flavors of mango and lychee.

Lychees were always easy to love, their perfume and sweetness made for a child's palate, and they offer forth abundant tactile pleasure. The carapace of the lychee is hard, bumpy, and red, with a puckery, tannic taste. Peel that away for the fruit — smooth, slippery, glowing white. Pop it in your mouth. It is so tender and full of juice, you barely have to chew — it gives itself up to you until at its center, you come to the smooth, oblong seed the color of cinnabar. Lychees are not to be eaten parsimoniously. They invite a blessed trance of eating until they are gone.

Mangoes were a harder sell to me as a child. As an uptight kid, I wanted everything tidy and symmetrical. There is nothing tidy about a mango. They'd fall with a thud from our tree in the backyard, exploding into a messy yuck. I would have been happy to leave them as a feast for the possums, who'd bore through them with their sharp teeth. Mangoes resembled possums, hanging down on long stems the way possums could hang from the tree by their tails. But one of my chores was to get to the mangoes and clean them up before they stained the deck. The sticky sap, with its whiff of turpentine, itched, put me in a sneezing fit, and made my eyelids swell until my eyes were slits.

There was no escaping them. Mangoes and avocados are to South Florida summer what zucchini is elsewhere in the country. No sooner would I recover from cleaning up the backyard than our neighbors would give their own mangoes to us — no, press them upon us unbidden.

You could count on a mango having a hairy, odd-shaped pit. That was the only sure thing about it. Sometimes a mango had fibers that would stick in your teeth, and sometimes it was slippery. A banana required no guesswork. It was always soft, sweet, unsurprising. But you could never tell what you were going to get with a mango. Well, no wonder; there are over four hundred varieties of mango, and a goodly number of them grow in South Florida.

I long ago outgrew my childhood mango allergy and aversion. You've got extras? I'm glad to take them off your hands. Mangoes have a sort of reptilian-looking rind that comes in sherbet colors — pale green, butter yellow, orange slouching toward red. It is inedible and must be peeled away, revealing the golden flesh inside. The fruit tastes of honey and peach, with a whispering of carrot. They're richer in vitamin C than oranges, crazy with potassium and beta-carotene, and just incredibly, delectably good.

To get at the goodness within, take a knife and gently score the mango in quarters. Don't try to cut through it — that funky pit will not allow you to. Just grab the top of each section and pull down. The skin will peel away from the flesh. Then slice, chop, or dice the mango, as you like. You can suck on that pit, albeit hairy and untidy in the extreme, and it will in no wise disappoint. It may, however, dribble a trail of golden juice down your shirt, an indelible reminder of your bliss.

There is a two-week window in July when both the lychees and mangoes are ripe and the air is heady with jasmine, real jasmine, the white blooms suddenly popping open under cover of darkness like the specter of a woman who appears only at night, dizzying the air with her perfume.

Breathe in the jasmine and eat the fruit now before it is gone, eat with abandon and without clothing, because it is so hot and both mangoes and lychees are so juicy. I've sacrificed more than one T-shirt to mango stains and have not regretted it. Lychees taught me pleasure, but mangoes remind me of the rewards of embracing my mess.

West Indian Mango Madness

Gorgeous, ripe summer fruit deserves to be eaten as is, without additives, frippery, or monkeying. No lycheetinis, no raspberry frappés, and no mango upside-down cakes. However, there are exceptions. Mangoes are your friends. During the assault of fruit when you can't keep pace with the glut, you can peel, slice, and freeze them for later. Or you can say what the hell and make this curry, which isn't really mad, but it's mango, which adds just the right sweet and tang to this island-inspired dish.

It's mild of spice, although you can ramp up the heat, and the whole thing comes together in a few minutes. Callaloo is better known elsewhere as amaranth, and if you know it at all, it's because of its tiny whole grains. In the Caribbean, it's beloved for its greens, emerald bright to brighten the spirit. If callaloo's not fresh and local, bok choy or napa cabbage is in season and glad to take its place.

West Indian Mango Madness

It's summer, so serve the madness more toward room temperature than flat-out hot off the stove. Pair with brown rice, Caribbean pigeon peas and rice, or roti or Flatbread from a Starter (page 214).

Serves 4

⅓ cup cashews
¼ cup whole wheat or chickpea flour or, if it's all you have,
    unbleached all-purpose flour
1½ teaspoons ground allspice
1½ teaspoons turmeric
Pinch of sea salt, plus more for seasoning
1 pound firm tofu
2 tablespoons canola or coconut oil
2 onions, thinly sliced
4 cloves garlic, minced
1 thumb-size piece fresh ginger, peeled and minced
½ jalapeño chili, minced (optional)
2 bunches callaloo, 2 bunches bok choy, or ½ napa
    cabbage, chopped into bite-size pieces
1 nice-size ripe mango, peeled and chopped
Juice of 1 or 2 limes
Sea salt and freshly ground pepper
1 bunch cilantro, coarsely chopped

Preheat oven to 350°F. Coarsely chop the cashews and place them in a shallow baking pan. Bake until golden brown, about 10 minutes.

In a shallow bowl, mix together the flour, ½ teaspoon of the all-spice, ½ teaspoon of the turmeric, and the pinch of sea salt.

Squeeze excess water from the tofu, blot dry with a kitchen towel, and cut into bite-size cubes. Working in batches, add the tofu cubes to the bowl and toss gently, until the tofu cubes are evenly dusted with the flour mixture.

In a large sauté pan (with straight sides, as opposed to a skillet, which has sloped sides), heat 1 tablespoon of the oil over medium-high heat.

Line a plate with paper towels and place near the stove. Carefully place about half the tofu cubes in the pan, with enough space so that the little guys aren't crowded. Cook until the tofu cubes get a nice little bit of crust on most sides, turning as needed with a spatula, about 9 to 10 minutes. Transfer the tofu to a plate or paper towel to absorb any extra oil. Repeat with the remaining tofu.

No need to wipe out the pan. Use it to heat the remaining 1 tablespoon oil over medium-high heat. Add the onions, garlic, ginger, jalapeño (if you like), and the remaining teaspoon each turmeric and allspice. Cook, stirring now and again, until the onions are golden from the turmeric, fragrant, and slightly tender, 5 to 8 minutes. Reduce the heat to medium, as needed, if the onions are sticking to the bottom of the pan.

Add your lovely chopped greens, a handful at a time, and cook until they just wilt, about 8 minutes for bok choy, just a minute or so for napa cabbage — callaloo's cook time is somewhere in the middle. Add the mango and lime juice and stir to combine.

Toss in the tofu and stir gently to heat through, about 4 to 5 minutes. Season with salt and pepper.

Stir in the cilantro and scatter the cashews on top.

Easy, fabulous.

GENTLE NUDGE *the* SEVENTH: TENDING — *and* HARVESTING — YOUR OWN GARDEN

Voltaire said we must tend our own gardens. He meant it's tough to change the world and it can get ugly and overwhelming out there, anyway. Be strategic, specific, use your energy to nurture your strengths. That, in turn, makes your own world better.

Voltaire was speaking in metaphor. These are days that call for action, not words, though. While you're tending your own metaphoric plot of ground, tend some real stuff. Grow some of what you eat.

As a teenage Goth, I got into gardening for the romance — Keats's Isabella watered her pot of basil with her tears (her lover's head was inside the urn; there were issues). My teenage metaphoric garden had unnaturally high yields of angst. But it turned out I could grow more productive things, not just basil, but arugula and tomatoes and collards and okra and peppers and broccoli. It felt weirdly empowering, providing a sense of Emersonian self-reliance along with the vegetables. I dialed down a little bit on the eyeliner.

Voltaire never said our gardens have to be big. Just growing a pot of herbs on a sunny windowsill will yield enough to spark up some salads and make you part of the growing process, a coaxer and creator of life. Growing gives you something from almost nothing. Nature is incredibly benevolent. I am not the dirt whisperer. My plants grow because they're in healthy soil and get the sun and water they need. Would that our own needs were so simple.

There is no better teacher than a garden — of any size. It reveals the rhythms of the earth. It shows how all its elements, from the seed to the soil to the sun, come together to produce what you eat in a minute.

It teaches humility. I don't kid myself. I may be growing vegetables, or trying to, but the earth is running this show, not me. I had big plans when I planted purslane — tomato and purslane salad, for one. The purslane had other ideas. Like not growing. The seeds, from a local organic farmer, sprouted. All very exciting. I made much over the seedlings, praising them mightily. Then they died. Too much sun? Not enough sun? Not enough water? Poor soil drainage? Poor self-esteem?

It does not help to yell at plants. It does not make them grow faster. Or at all. Growth happens as it does, if it does — over time. I hate this. I like the point of things, the result, the harvest, more than the process. But I am learning.

Growing teaches the sweet rewards of patience. I try to think of time as the secret ingredient in cooking, the necessary but natural input in the soil, the trick that turns hey-how-are-ya into true friendship, the magic that makes everything come together. This was the lesson I harvested instead of purslane.

If I have crop failure, it's annoying, disappointing. But it reminds me just how dependent we are on the earth and how grateful I am for true organic farmers who grow the bulk of what I eat. It teaches gratitude, to cultivate a little reverence along with your radicchio. It makes me more grateful for the miracle of fresh, ripe tomatoes.

Their names alone delight — Cherokee Purple, Mr. Stripey, Pink Ping Pong. They're heirlooms from local farmers and gifted gardener friends. As *heirloom* suggests, they've been bred over generations and passed down with love, recognized for the treasures they are. They bear but the slightest resemblance to the basic beefsteak tomatoes in your supermarket, green gassed and baseball hard. I'm tired of tasteless tomatoes, tired of our increasingly one-variety-is-all-you-get world. Why shy from variety? Why deny ourselves flavor?

My heirlooms grow leafy and leggy inside a three-foot tomato cage. They are smaller than supermarket tomatoes and not always pinup perfect, but they're tender, juicy, yielding, warm from the sun, tempting your hands, your mouth. They have give, they have heft, they have chi.

Bring your face to them. Breathe in. Tomato plants give off a scent some call astringent. I call it sexual musk. Fresh tomatoes make you want to bring them directly to your mouth, to touch their thin membrane of skin with your lips, to enter the fruit with your teeth. It is not for nothing the French have called the tomato *pomme d'amour* — "apple of love."

This may be other than what Voltaire had in mind when he wrote of tending your own garden, but he was a Frenchman, after all. He would understand. At least he'd deign to have some salad.

Summer Tomato Salad with Za'atar

This summer salad relies on fresh, ripe tomatoes and little else. It comes together superfast. Find za'atar, a spice blend of sumac, thyme, and sesame seeds, in most Middle Eastern markets. It adds a haunting, elusive flavor — the taste of wisdom. Should the za'atar itself prove elusive to obtain, the salad will still be bright and happy without it — though perhaps not as wise.

Nice with a fluffy, whole grainy dish like the Judeo-Christian Barley Salad (page 69).

Serves 4

3 gorgeous ripe tomatoes, chopped, or 3 cups grape
    tomatoes, halved, or a mix of the two
Juice of 2 or 3 lemons
3 tablespoons olive oil
1 fennel bulb, halved (if large) and thinly sliced
2 scallions, chopped
1 handful kalamata olives, pitted
1 handful fresh mint
1 tablespoon za'atar
Sea salt and freshly ground pepper

First, grow your tomatoes.

Okay, that step is optional.

In a small bowl, whisk together the lemon juice and olive oil until emulsified.

Add the fennel, tomatoes, scallions, and olives and toss to combine. Gently fold in the mint and the za'atar. Season with salt and pepper.

Enjoy at room temperature.

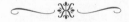

INTENSE HEAT

I don't associate fasting with greater spiritual insight. Benjamin would prefer not to associate with fasting at all. But I fast at Yom Kippur, the Jewish day of atonement, which falls late in the harvest season — one shot, one day, and you're good to go. It reminds me to appreciate the simple things I take for granted — a good, strong cup of joe in the morning, a fresh, gentle pear at lunch.

But, you know, it's a single day off your feed; it is not a marathon fast like Lent or Ramadan. Ramadan takes its name from *al-ramad* — intense heat. It happens during the ninth month of the Islamic calendar, the hottest month of the year — usually corresponding to July. It's thirty days of prayer and fasting from dawn to dusk, a time of returning to yourself and your family, of pledging your faith anew.

We are too easily distracted by silly worldly things. We always have been. It's the way we're made. Two hundred years before iPhones and reality shows, Wordsworth wrote: "The world is too much with us; late and soon, / Getting and spending, we lay waste our powers: / Little we see in Nature that is ours; / We have given our hearts away, a sordid boon!"

I would have lost the exclamation point at the end, but the poem's meaning resonates. I'm fully guilty of distraction, of making myself crazy over nothing. The ritual of Ramadan appeals to me, and summer is the time to do it — it makes for a kind of bikram penance. Hot weather takes a whack at our appetites and burns away our less pleasant qualities, boiling us down to the essence of ourselves. At least that was my experience in Morocco.

Most of the Sahara is what's known as stone desert, miles and miles of flat, dusty, stone-pocked, blasted lunar landscape. Benjamin and I had been driving all day on the rocky, roadless surface, reaching, by nightfall, a *ksar*, a compound made of mud, standing all by itself, miles from anywhere at all.

In the dark, the wind blew, the sand stung us. We knocked at the thick, arched wooden door, and after a time, a woman in robes admitted us. Inside, within the *ksar*'s high walls, the wind stopped, the air became still and silent. She showed us to our bare room, then to the central courtyard, strung with colored lights and lit with lanterns. We should come out when we were ready, she said. She would bring us dinner.

In Marrakech, we'd stayed at a *riad*, a traditional Moroccan home built around a central courtyard. Our room was at one end, next to the kitchen, from which came heady aromas. I tiptoed by and watched two staff women at work. They were easy together in the kitchen, with its elaborate black-and-white tiled floor and not a single modern appliance in sight. They were working, but talking, too, and laughing, dancing, singing — and sometimes ululating — to music. People cook together, friends and extended family — that's what they do. And there is always something to be done in the kitchen, so after beating back shyness, I joined them. I picked up a knife — duller than mine at home but capable of chopping carrots, onions, and zucchini for a vegetable tagine, Morocco's famed slow-simmering stew. One cook steamed and fluffed couscous. Her friend flipped semolina griddle bread. The only Arabic phrase I knew was, "Please, special price? For me?" It didn't matter. We could gesture, we could smile, we could nod to create a richly flavored meal and, to me, a richer day.

In Fez, we had gone shopping in the souks, where vendors displayed barrows brimming with thistly wild artichokes; bins of lustrous purple eggplants; baskets of fresh, fragrant mint; figs spilling their seeds and secrets; pyramids of dried apricots, furled like ears; pillar-size jars of spices; burlap bags filled with grains and dried beans; and at the local butcher's stall, the head of a camel. The rest of him was missing.

In the desert, though, miles from anywhere, including the nearest market, local food takes on a different meaning. Nothing in the Sahara is local except dates and olives. In one of the great cosmic coincidences, though, they are among the most sustaining foods. They're what you're first served at Iftar, the breaking of the fast at the end of day during Ramadan, and they were what our robed hostess set down in front of us. Then she brought out a ceramic cooking vessel with a conical lid. This, too, is called a tagine.

She lifted the lid, revealing not a vegetable stew, but a tumble of rice and a perfumed steam that promised something more. The rice was studded with toasted almonds, heady with saffron and olive oil, and, every now and again, never when you'd expect it, you'd come to another sliver of date. Tender, crunchy, simple but somehow thrilling, it was made entirely of pantry staples and a certain amount of genius. It was the perfect thing at journey's end, like being enveloped in the arms of a friend.

I can't quite give you the whole Saharan experience, but this rice might get you close. I have added some lentils for protein and interest. They're appropriately shelf stable, too. I would also like to throw in some green vegetables but, in order to be true to the original, have held off. Though it pairs very nicely with the broccoli recipe later in this chapter (see page 145), Broccoli with Lemon and Mint (Broccoli for Beginners). I'm just saying.

Rice in the Sahara

Serves 4 to 6

½ cup slivered almonds

3 cups Stone Soup (see page 84) or other vegetable broth or
    water

1 cup brown rice

2 tablespoons olive oil

1 onion, sliced

Pinch of saffron

½ cup red lentils
1 cinnamon stick
1 teaspoon ground allspice
3 dried Medjool dates, chopped
Sea salt and freshly ground pepper

Preheat the oven to 375°F. Pour the almonds in a shallow oven-proof pan and toast until they just turn golden and are fragrant, 8 to 10 minutes. Transfer the almonds to a small bowl to cool.

In a medium saucepan, bring 2 cups of the vegetable broth to a boil over high heat. Add the rice, cover, and reduce the heat to low. Simmer just until the rice absorbs the liquid and leans toward tenderness, about 30 minutes. (It will continue cooking later.) Remove from the heat and let cool. (The rice can be stored in an airtight container in the refrigerator for a day or two; bring to room temperature before proceeding with the recipe.)

In a large skillet, heat the oil over medium-high heat. Add the onion and stir until evenly coated. Cover, reduce the heat to low, and cook about 20 minutes. The onion will still be pale and will have thrown off quite a lot of liquid. This is good. Add the saffron and raise the heat to medium.

Add the red lentils to the onions and stir to combine. Add the remaining 1 cup broth, cover again, and continue cooking. Red lentils cook speedily — 10 to 15 minutes. Check them after 12 minutes. They should be pale rosy and tender, not mushy.

Add the cinnamon stick to the onion-lentil mixture, and stir in the allspice, cooked rice, and dates. Season with plenty of salt and pepper.

Heat over medium heat for a few minutes, stirring to combine, until heated through. Just before serving, stir in the toasted almonds for a nice crunch.

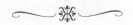

Afterward, we slept. When the hostess knocked to wake us, it was still dark, just after three in the morning. I dressed, splashed water on my face, brushed my hair, and put on a swipe of lipstick. I wanted to look nice.

We opened the door into...an abyss. The desert at night is not merely dark; it is cold and so black it seems to create a vacuum. The stars blaze above, stolen diamonds, but they do not light your way. You cannot see out, you cannot see down. To walk, I would have to go on faith.

A beam of light also helps. A man stood, holding a flashlight — our Berber guide, swathed in blue robes.

"Come," he said. "Your camels are ready."

I'd put on lipstick — a shade called desert rose — for the camels. I wanted them to like me, as I knew I would love them. They knelt in the sand, saddled with blankets. I fell to my knees to greet them.

Perhaps it was the wrong shade of lipstick. Like our spare, elegant guide, they seemed impervious to the wind, the sand, us. But they tolerated us when we got on. When the guide gave the command, they rose onto their front legs, pitching us backward. Then they rose onto their hind legs; we all wobbled, got our bearings, and proceeded out of the stone desert and into the dunes.

We trekked for hours. Our guide did not say much. He did not have to. The only sound was the muffled thudding of our camels' hooves on the sand. The blackness of the night gave way to pearly first light, and the dunes surrounding us revealed themselves — rose and honey and salmon colored, an ocean of sand, vast and alive, blown high by the wind into sensuous peaks and sweeps.

This sand was not the sand that had pelted us outside the *ksar* the night before. It was entirely other, so fine as to be almost liquid, like satin on my skin. The dunes' surface was already growing warm from the sun, but I plunged my hands down into the sand below, where it felt cool to the touch.

We sat, watching the sun rise above the dunes, first a piercing red light above the sand, then a band of it, and then the entire sun rising as though in a hurry. Why hurry? There were only the wide stretches and scoops of sand; what novelist Paul Bowles called the sheltering sky above; and us. I felt Bowles's definition of magic, "a secret connection between the world of nature and the consciousness of man, a hidden but direct passage that bypassed the mind."

The desert rang with primeval magic. We breathed its air, full of secrets that would reveal themselves, if only you would wait.

I waited. The desert told me one.

You need nothing, it said. You are fine.

"We go," our guide said.

Go? Why would we go? I wanted to stay. Forever. Fez, Marrakech, Miami, what did I need with any of it? I wanted to disappear into the dunes like Kit Morseby in Bowles's *The Sheltering Sky*. Having a surreal and sexual nervous breakdown like hers was negotiable.

"It is hot," our guide said.

So it was. In the midst of my ecstatic experience, I had somehow failed to notice. Likewise I had not noticed Benjamin and I were covered with desert dust. Our guide, however, was immaculate. Berber robes and headgear aren't a fashion statement. They make sense. So did water. I drank. And drank.

We mounted our camels; they lurched to their feet and led us out of the dunes and back to where the desert wore down to stone. It was still morning, but the sun's heat was a power, as absolute as the night, or an ocean, or an ocean of sand. And out in the desert, there is no escaping it, no cover, no shade. I felt stunned by the sun and as dry and gray as the endless stone desert. I felt humbled by the Sahara, beholden to it, at its mercy.

We plodded on. Then I saw something odd. Something green and scrubby in the rocks, as though the Sahara had grown an unfortunate soul patch. Then there were lots of green things pushing through, then whole ribbons of green erupting from the rocks and sand. I wondered if I was hallucinating and then, ever given to extremes, if I was somehow dying of typhus like *The Sheltering Sky*'s Port Moresby.

I cleared my parched throat. "Is this...are these...*shrubs?*"

The Sahara's surface is dry, our guide explained, but water flows beneath, close to the surface. When it comes close enough, things grow.

Then he smiled. For the first time. It transformed him, turning him from stony to vital and alive.

"Where there is water," he said, "there is life." He called it an oasis.

I call it a miracle. And you know, I'm not one to bandy the word around.

a BOWL of WELL-BEING

It is not always possible to run away to the desert. Who has the time? And there's always the risk you'll have too much of a *Sheltering Sky* experience. But a little heat, a little magic — these are worthwhile things, and a pot of harira supplies both.

Like dates and olives, harira is a Ramadan tradition, deeply restorative at the end of a day of fasting and repentance, making use of a riot of fresh summer vegetables, like tomatoes and zucchini. The result is something greater than the sum of its parts.

Every family makes its own version of harira. It is entirely forgiving, allowing you to add more of this or that. You can make it elegant with a pinch of saffron or *ras el hanout*, a mystical blend of spices and peppers and flowers, or you can make it simple and straightforward and still come away with a fair amount of enchantment. The only must-have is yeast. This is traditional for harira, giving it some oomph and thickness and a mild fermenty kick. After that first taste — where you go, hmm, odd — it becomes addictive. I've since seen harira recipes with lamb, with chicken, with eggs. I haven't seen many plant-based versions like mine, though.

Harira somehow satisfies but does not stuff you. Maybe it's the yeast. Certainly it's the yeast that lifts this soup of summer vegetables from everyday to exotic. It lifts my spirits, too. When I make harira, I like to think of the women in my Marrakech *riad* making it for their own families, and somehow, someone in the desert enjoying it, too. What's the point in having magic if you can't whisk a pot of soup to someone when you like?

Excellent during Ramadan, when it's served at dusk, along with olives and dates, to break the daylong fast, it is quite the thing any time of year. Enjoy it nontraditionally when the weather is bitter and cold or you are bitter and have a cold. It's energizing, restorative, warming. It is well-being in a bowl.

Harira

Serves 8

2 tablespoons olive oil

1 large onion, chopped

1 teaspoon turmeric

3 zucchini or yellow squash or a mix of the two, chopped

2 red bell peppers, chopped

2 stalks celery, chopped

Pinch of saffron or *ras el hanout* (optional but very nice)

One 28-ounce can diced tomatoes or 4 gorgeous ripe
   tomatoes, chopped

One 15-ounce can chickpeas, rinsed and drained

6 cups Stone Soup (see page 84) or other vegetable broth

1 small handful whole wheat vermicelli or angel hair pasta,
   broken into bite-size pieces

1 tablespoon active dry yeast dissolved in ¼ cup warm
   vegetable broth or water

Juice of 1 or 2 lemons

Sea salt and freshly ground pepper

1 handful fresh cilantro, chopped

Lemon wedges for serving (optional)

In a large stockpot, heat the olive oil over medium-high heat. Add the onion and turmeric. Cook, stirring, until the onion softens and turns golden, a few minutes. Add the zucchini, red bell peppers, celery, and, if you've got it, the saffron or *ras el hanout*. Cook, stirring occasionally, until the vegetables become tender, 5 to 8 minutes more.

Stir in the tomatoes, chickpeas, and broth. Reduce the heat to medium-low and simmer, uncovered, 45 minutes to 1 hour.

Add the broken pasta, yeast mixture, and lemon juice and stir to combine. Continue cooking 3 to 5 minutes more, until the angel hair softens, stirring occasionally. Season with sea salt and pepper. Just before serving, stir in the cilantro.

Serve with extra lemon wedges, if desired.

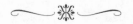

GENTLE NUDGE *the* EIGHTH:
STOCKED *and* STOKED

Every so often, Benjamin likes to open the doors to our kitchen cupboard. It puts him into a rapturous trance. It is, he says, a thing of wonder that'd do an alchemist proud, with bags of spices, grains, and seeds, mysterious bottles and jars filled with bright-colored oils and amber syrups, all spilling forth — and sometimes spilling out. I may not be tidy, but I am prepared. Having a well-stocked larder is useful, whether you're in the Sahara or San Francisco. It means you'll always have what it takes to put together a magical meal. Magic, after all, needs a little help. Your starter supply might set you back twenty-five dollars. Aside from the olive oil, these ingredients add no fat to your food, but all add plenty of energy and nutrition, plus the makings for a year's worth of diverse and vibrant meals. A whole year's worth. Come on, you can blow that much at Starbucks without even working up an espresso-induced sweat.

The Basics

LEGUMES. Protein-rich, fiberrific beans, like lentils, garbanzos, black beans, and cute little white cannellini. Having a few cans of beans means you can have a meal in minutes. Dried beans are cheaper and have an indefinite shelf life. Why choose? Keep a few of each on hand.

WHOLE GRAINS. Grains with their nutrient-rich kernel and fiber-rich bran intact. Once written off as peasant food, they're now recognized as dietary darlings, and we're coming to appreciate them for what they always have been — delicious, each with its own unique flavor and texture. Get the ones you know, like oatmeal and brown rice, then step out and try bitsy amaranth, nutty barley, nuttier buckwheat. And quinoa, the quick-cooking ancient grain that's so fun to say; it has a subtle taste of wild fields, and the tiny grains feel like bubbles in the mouth.

EXTRA-VIRGIN OLIVE OIL. This is the oil our bodies like to process. It's rich in cancer-beating antioxidants, with a high smoke point, which makes it great for cooking, and a silky fruitiness. Extra-virgin means it's made from the first pressing of the olives. It has lower acidity and more antioxidants than other olive-oil grades. It's elegant, madly versatile, and just a touch gilds a dish. Homer called it liquid gold. I'm talking the Homer who wrote the *Iliad* and the *Odyssey*, not Homer Simpson, who has his own views on food. Please remember he is a cartoon character.

SEA SALT. Why can sea salt cost anywhere from three to ten dollars a pop, when a big ol' last-you-forever canister of the supermarket kind only sets you back fifty cents? Because sea salt offers the one-two punch of better flavor and better nutrition. Table salt is refined, with its natural minerals processed out and anticaking agents added in. Sea salt has none of table salt's burn or bitterness and is naturally mineral rich. It has a mildness on the palate, almost like a spice unto itself. It comes in a whole rainbow of colors, including crunchy pink Himalayan salt and French sel gris — gray salt. I'm especially crazy about Maldon salt, from Essex, England, with magnificent white crystal flakes that dazzle the tongue and make for fun crunching. Pricey, but so vibrant, you need only a little.

WHOLE PEPPERCORNS. The pepper in your pepper shaker was probably ground back in the last ice age. It's so dusty and bland, it'll last you till the next ice age because you rarely use it. Give your mouth some fun. Whole peppercorns are like pearls that release their fullness and spark when crushed. Freshly cracked pepper adds not just heat but depth of flavor. It beats the panties off the old ground stuff. Go wild. Buy a pepper mill, too.

The Brushstrokes

Legumes, whole grains, olive oil, sea salt, and pepper will take you far. They're your survival staples. Very nice, but you deserve more. What about thrills and delights? What about full frontal flavor? These culinary treasures are to bland food as an artist's palette is to a blank canvas.

CONDIMENTS

You don't need seventy kinds of mustard and forty kinds of pickles. Start with the big three — an earthy, grainy mustard; a rich, fermented soy sauce; and a syrupy, aged balsamic vinegar. They add depth and dimension to food, but no fat or calories.

Ready to upgrade? Ingredients that were impossible to get a few years ago are now on market shelves or just a click away on the Internet. I'm in love with sweet-tart pomegranate molasses and the layers of salty, tangy flavors of preserved lemons. All these ingredients dazzle with flavors vibrant and unique. Like love, they can't be faked. Unlike love, they can be bought.

SPICES

Spices are the dried, ground bark or seeds of plants. Herbs are the green, leafy parts. Herbs tend to be cooling, while spices are warming. Think of the difference between anise seed and tarragon. Both have licorice notes, but anise, a spice, has a gentle coziness to it, while fresh tarragon leaves provide a light licorice lift. Jarred dried spices last up to two years if kept out of the light, so stock up. Dried herbs, on the other hand, are just sad-making.

They'll do in a pinch but, at best, will remind you of their live, fresh incarnation. Experiment and educate your palate. Find the seasonings you like. Use them generously. Try new ones. The spices without which I would not care to live include the following.

CARDAMOM. Rich, mellow cardamom is the star of chai, India's fragrant spiced tea (see recipe, page 195), Arabic coffee, and Dutch and African recipes, too. It's not cheap, costing right up there with saffron and vanilla, but it's an aphrodisiac according to *Tales of a Thousand and One Nights*. It's pretty sexy stuff. Less mythic, more scientific findings show it aids digestion and has a mighty congestion-busting phytochemical.

CHILIES. The big bang of spices. And the bang is capsaicin, a heart-healthy antioxidant that blasts cholesterol and triglycerides. Chilies are loaded with vitamins A, C, and E. They stimulate your heart and circulation the way they stimulate your palate and sinuses. They fire up foods from corn bread to the beany, spicy mélange that bears their name — chili. How spicy is up to you — and the Scoville scale. The Scoville scale rates the heat of every chili pepper, from the barely-there bell pepper, which has a rating of zero, to the incendiary, legendary ghost chili, which has a rating of over a million. I love 'em all, especially three winning dried red chili peppers from Turkey — Aleppo, with its gentle heat; its sassier sister, Marash; and darker, sharper Urfa, with its deliciously guttural name.

CINNAMON. Antimicrobial, anti-inflammatory, and circulation improving, cinnamon aids your respiratory and digestive systems. Not only does this warming, sweet spice add a note of grace to fruits and desserts, but studies indicate that just a quarter teaspoon a day (a dash in your cappuccino, on your oatmeal, or on a fresh peach) can help lower blood-sugar levels.

CORIANDER. Coriander is kin to cilantro — in fact, they began life as the same plant. Coriander is the seeds; cilantro is the leaves. Anti-inflammatory, antibiotic, and a cholesterol killer, this is a superversatile spice, rich in vitamin C. The Egyptians embraced it five thousand years ago for both its healthful properties and its sultry notes of citrus and sage. It's belonged to Arab cuisine ever since, as well as to the cuisines of Mexico, the Caribbean, India, Asia, and Morocco.

CUMIN. This earthy Egyptian spice naturally contains iron for immunity and stimulates digestion. It also zaps potential nasties thanks to its antimicrobial properties. It may help fight cancer as well. All this, and it's a must-have for cuisines from the Middle East to Mexico.

GINGER. This dried, ground rhizome (great word, means "root-stock") earns its age-old reputation as a stomach settler and a puri-fier. It has cholesterol-lowering, artery-degunking antioxidants, and antifungal, blood-clotting, and cancer-whacking properties. You can't make Asian or Indian food without it. Or gingerbread.

TURMERIC. The other rhizome on the list and the golden spice in every curry powder known to man. It's valued not just for its gentle heat, but for its anti-inflammatory powers, and may be a player in combating Alzheimer's. Research indicates it breaks up plaque deposits in the brain. It's integral to Indian food and makes mustard yellow.

These spices complement each other in recipes and in your body, too. Chilies' circulatory power allows for better turmeric absorption. A hot infusion of ginger, cinnamon, and cardamom eases both respiratory and gastric woes. It's like a divine meant-to-be.

RECIPE *for* DISASTER

I excel at denial. I'm not proud of it; but it's a coping mechanism, and it's served me well in times of crisis. I've even been able to shrug off a hurricane. It might have been on the weatherman's radar, but it wasn't on mine. We hadn't gotten a hurricane in years, and Miami never got them in August. Why worry? I was more focused on meeting a story deadline and meeting a friend for a little fun. I needed some fun.

Dismissing a major weather event was one thing. Harder was denying the fact that Benjamin and I were in a spot of bad weather ourselves.

Our first two years of married life, we'd lived in Tokyo in a little apartment. Benjamin was there for work; I was there for romance — a new husband, a new life, a new country. It was the best kind of adventure, being in love, playing house, traveling Asia, making things up as we went along. In-laws and responsibility existed in another time zone.

Then we came back to Miami, where each of our favorite grandmothers died within months of each other. We rented another apartment; I worked days to put Benjamin through grad school courses he took at night. We barely saw each other but soldiered on with a sense of duty now for the future — not my favorite sense. He passed the CPA exam his first time out, in one heroic go, and got a job with an accounting firm, and we bought a house.

These are good things, things you strive for, yes? Here was our reward, our harvest, the fruits of our labor. It all accreted on me like weights. I felt left behind, lonely. Benjamin had grown up, I hadn't, and we were never going to have fun again. The whole world gave way beneath me. I had no idea where I was going. And oh, good, we were going to have a hurricane, too.

I did not know how I was going to survive being stuck in this house with this husband. Oh, they were both nice enough; I was the problem. I was bratty, snappish, and moody. I could barely stand myself.

Further proof of my freakishness — I am not particularly into chocolate. But I'm not stupid, okay? I needed dark chocolate's antioxidants and mood modifiers. If I was going to manage this hurricane at all, a cake would be necessary. Some vegan chocolate cakes are good, some decidedly not, but most comprise arcane ingredients like xanthan gum. I'm sorry, I still don't know what that is.

I took a mental-health break to look through Laurie Colwin's wonderful book *More Home Cooking*. I love her cozy way of giving you a recipe for something simple and comforting, something you want to eat right now, and happily, you can because it's made with things you have on hand. Combined, though, these ingredients become greater than the sum of their parts. This not only yields you something worth eating; it makes you feel like you've executed a magic trick. If I couldn't have fun, at least I'd have chocolate cake.

I did some vegan ingredient swapping for Colwin's recipe and came up with a cake that's quick, easy, pantry friendly, almost guilt-free, and totally vegan — and still provides a mind-blowing chocolate experience.

Vegan Chocolate Cake

Serves 8 to 10

½ cup canola oil, plus more for the cake pan
1¾ cups unbleached all-purpose flour
¾ cup unsweetened cocoa powder
1 teaspoon baking soda
1 cup evaporated cane sugar
1 cup unsweetened almond milk
2 teaspoons apple cider vinegar
2 teaspoons pure vanilla extract
Powdered sugar for garnish

Preheat the oven to 350°F. Lightly oil a 9-inch round cake pan.

In a large bowl, sift together the flour, cocoa, and baking soda. Stir in the sugar.

In a small bowl, stir together the almond milk and vinegar. It will curdle; don't fret. Stir in the ½ cup canola oil and the vanilla.

Gently stir the wet ingredients into the flour-cocoa mixture until just combined and it all coalesces into a dark, thick batter.

Pour into the prepared cake pan. Bake until the fragrance of chocolate wafts through the room, about 30 minutes. You can also give the cake a gentle poke with a finger; it should spring back when baked through.

All it needs is a dusting of powdered sugar.

The cake can be wrapped well and stored in the refrigerator for several days; bring to room temperature just before serving.

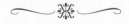

So I had the cake. But even I couldn't deny that the whirling computer-generated graphic the meteorologists were calling Hurricane Andrew was bearing down on Miami. And the local television weather folk, normally so smiley and composed beneath their pancake makeup, were starting to blink, stutter, and sweat. Whatever else I might be dealing with or denying would have to wait.

I went about doing the normal hurricane prep, laying in candles and canned food, taking in the plants and patio furniture, all the while singing the R.E.M. ditty "It's the End of the World as We Know It (and I Feel Fine)."

Just as the winds started to kick in, Benjamin lowered our blinds and latched them, turning our house from breezy, open, and flooded with sunshine to dark and close, the set of Sartre's *No Exit*.

Low-pressure system outside, high-pressure system inside. No wonder Benjamin got socked with a major headache. He wisely took to bed.

I didn't. I read, paced, drank tea, made ice, picked up a book, put it down, watched the weather reports. The stations kept running footage of palm trees battered by the wind, meteorologists in yellow rain slickers squinting through the rain at the camera. This was before hurricane predicting became state of the art. South Florida only realized the power and path of Hurricane Andrew, a category 4 storm, as it hit.

It knocked out our electricity by ten o'clock. The phone line went dead an hour later. With the windows shuttered, I couldn't see out, couldn't see what the hurricane was doing. But I could hear it. I did not know wind could scream. It keened like a banshee around us all night long, and it was all I could do not to scream right along with it. Gusts smacked the house and shook the foundation till I thought we would twist and spin up and away like Dorothy's house in *The Wizard of Oz*.

And then all fell quiet. The storm passed by morning. This was the moment for Benjamin and me to turn and embrace each other, grateful we were still alive. We didn't. But together, we ventured from our dark, shuttered house into sunshine. The sky was clear, the air freshly laundered. As I looked up, it was as if the hurricane had never been. But down here on earth, fallen trees — some as high as homes — blocked the road; power lines were down; weird bits of debris — shattered roof tiles, jagged, splintered tree limbs, shreds of clothing, a single hubcap — were strewn all over the block.

The thing is, as bad as a hurricane is, you don't know how bad until afterward. This happened at a time of few cell phones or laptops. Discovering how friends and relatives were, how the rest of Miami had done, was piecemeal and protracted, a slow, painful relay of information from person to person. My aunt had no roof and extensive flooding. A friend had lost home, car, belongings, everything. Houses were smashed along one southwestern stretch of the city, as though by a cranky giant. Citywide infrastructure was demolished, too.

It is hard to get up a good oh-woe-is-me-am-I-getting-what-I-need-in-my-relationship thing going at times like this. There were bigger issues.

After just a few unplugged hours, you realize how big a part electricity plays in our daily lives, how brilliantly we use it to insulate ourselves, how vulnerable we are without it. It didn't take long to feel the full force of the subtropics. This was August. It was hot. And humid. And humbling. Within hours, everything felt sticky and saturated, including us. In these ideal hothouse conditions, mold and mildew blossomed on every surface. Food promptly started to rot in the refrigerator. Ice melted before our eyes, and there was no telling when we'd get more.

Junk food consumption spikes at times like these. The first time anyone bothered documenting this was after the September 11 World Trade Center attacks. The phenom is called terror eating, when you've had enough and take to bed — or scurry beneath it — with corn dogs and Pop-Tarts and tell the world to go to hell.

It is not a time you think of having a party. Yet our house was central, still standing, and, given the condition of the roads, relatively easy to get to. So the night after the hurricane, friends, family, neighbors, and a few strays gathered here. And I was glad. We all needed to be close, as hot and sticky as it was.

This does not mean we were perky. I was a zombified version of myself, and the people who came that night were no better. We were overwhelmed, haggard, ashen, and a bit on the ripe side. Some showed up tearful, others were angry, but everyone came and surrendered the bits and bobs of food they'd brought from home, food as tired and sorry as we were. I've seen more and peppier produce when I served at a soup kitchen. Even with everyone chipping in, dinner for ten would be a challenge. We had no oven, stove top, refrigerator, or coherent menu; I had no coherent brain. But we are a species of adaptation, whether we want to be or not. When all else fails, there is pasta.

Benjamin corralled everyone out back and fired up the gas grill. I set a big pot of water on top. And waited. After half an hour, we got something approaching a boil. After another half hour, the spaghetti had cooked to just a shade shy of al dente, and I was one click from despair. It would have to do. I took the pot off and drained off the pasta by holding a colander over a patch of dirt, saving some of the precious starchy cooking water for the sauce. Benjamin took everyone's donated meat and threw it on the grill. Our friends and family staggered around him.

I took the drained pasta inside. The tile floor, like my bare feet, sweated. Outside, the daylight was fading. Inside, it was dark. This is something you tend to forget in a city so in love with electricity that the streetlights blot out the stars at night. But take away power, and when the sun sets, it really sets. Oh, sure, there are the pretty bits when the sun fades, the light plays golden, and the sky goes all art-deco pastel, but then two minutes later, bam, it's black.

Alone in the kitchen, I lit a few candles to see by and chopped up the vegetables already wilting without refrigeration. I tossed them in a skillet with a glug of olive oil and gave them a stir and sauté over the Sterno stove — a flimsy little cardboard-and-metal stand erected over a can of flammable goo that provided some heat as well as noxious fumes. I held my breath. Then I sacrificed my last two lemons and squeezed them into the vegetables — my favorite way to zing up food. One lemon was so soft and tired, my thumb went right through it. I burst into tears.

A small, jewellike, rational part of me knew it was wrong to have survived a hurricane only to be defeated by a lemon. The rest of me told the rational part of me to shut up.

I addressed the universe. "Can't one frigging thing go right? Is that too much to ask?"

Apparently, it was. Because a few minutes later, a weird light began making its jerky way into the house. A break-in? A poltergeist? Sterno hallucination? Aneurysm? All inconvenient options right now. I went from sweaty to cold-sweaty.

Benjamin called out, "Ellen? Where are you?"

"*Paris*," I shouted. "I'm in Paris. I'm having a wonderful time, thanks. I'm in the *kitchen* — what did you think?"

He stood in the kitchen doorway, holding a flashlight, the source of my light, a tall man casting a taller shadow.

"I heard your voice. I thought something was —" He broke off. "I missed you." Or maybe he said, "I miss you."

I could not for the life of me imagine why. I would divorce myself if I could.

It was too hot for a tantrum, too hot to cry, but I started blubbing about the lemon, the hurricane, us. He grabbed me in a clumsy hug. It was too hot for hugs. I dropped the wooden spoon and threw both arms around him.

Then Benjamin, my guardian angel with a category 4 headache, shone the flashlight beam into the pot as I gave the pasta a last toss. He lit enough candles for a high mass, set them around the dining-room table, and called everyone in to eat.

We sat around the table, eating or not, the candles melting into mush, the flickering light casting monstrous shadows, the open windows bringing no relief of a breeze. The night and the tangle of fallen trees enclosed us all like a witch's enchantment.

Someone knocked at the door. I screamed. Benjamin did the more conventional and useful thing — he opened the door. There, in the darkness, stood a friend holding up a dripping bag, the last bag of ice in the city of Miami. He came in, handed over the ice, and pulled up a chair. We toasted him with refreshed drinks and spirits; he ate the rest of the pasta.

I brought out the chocolate cake. Even those who'd been too miserable for dinner sat up at the sight of dessert. We divvied up the cake among us.

In the candlelight's unsteady glow, Benjamin and I looked at each other from opposite ends of the table. Our problems were still going to be there. But we were here, with our friends and our family, in our house that was built to last. Maybe we were built to last, too. I'm not saying we all felt lucky, spared, saved. We felt okay. We felt we'd survived. In desperate times, that's a good first step.

It's a tricky first step, too. I tend to find hope as elusive as an ice cube in August — I have it, and then I don't. The big, cosmic lessons we each need to learn are the ones quickest forgotten — memory card full. But I have to start somewhere. Sometimes, it starts with making dinner.

I don't make this pasta often. I can be superstitious enough to think it invites calamity. I make it when I'm tapped out. And I'm always glad. It is not showy and is of no particular cultural or culinary tradition, other than necessity. But it's soothing, simple, and reminds me that even in disaster, there are shimmering moments of generosity and forgiveness and hope. Sometimes there's spaghetti, too.

When-All-Else-Fails Pasta (a.k.a. Ten-Minute Pasta with Zucchini, Tomatoes, and Chickpeas)

This recipe relies on vegetable workhorses (if that's not a mixed metaphor) like zucchini, tomatoes, and chickpeas. Also welcome — any and all herbs and any green vegetables in your fridge or freezer. Give us your tired broccoli, your poor freezer-burned peas. Add them to the pasta. The only semi-arcane ingredient is nutritional yeast. It is not necessary, but do not scoff at it. Rich in vitamin B_{12}, nutritional yeast is a vegan's best friend. It could be yours, too. Cheesy-tasting, dairy-free, and shelf-stable, it's a nice thing when your real cheese is sporting a blue fuzz of mold.

Serves 8 to 10 (you can halve the recipe if you like, in which case it serves a more seemly 4 to 5)

2 tablespoons olive oil
4 cloves garlic, minced
1 or 2 pinches red pepper flakes
4 zucchini, chopped
4 tomatoes, chopped, or one 28-ounce can diced tomatoes
Any extra vegetables you have on hand, chopped
    (optional)
Two 15-ounce cans chickpeas, rinsed and drained
1 pound whole wheat spaghetti or angel hair pasta
Juice of 2 lemons
Any stray bits of fresh herbs, chopped (optional)
¼ cup nutritional yeast (optional, but excellent)
Sea salt and freshly ground pepper

In a large skillet, heat the oil over medium-high heat. Add the garlic, red pepper flakes, and zucchini. Cook, stirring occasionally, until the garlic turns golden, the pepper flakes sizzle, and the zucchini softens, about 5 minutes.

Add the tomatoes and their juice, and any extra chopped vegetables you're in need of using up. Stir and cook for another few minutes until the mixture comes together as a nice, simple pan sauce. Stir in the chickpeas. Reduce the heat to medium, stirring occasionally, while in another large pot, you boil the pasta according to the package directions.

Drain the pasta, reserving ½ cup of the pasta cooking water, and return the cooked pasta to the large pot. Pour the zucchini-and-tomato mixture over the pasta and toss until the pasta is evenly coated in the sauce. Add the lemon juice and, if desired, some of the reserved pasta water for the ideal sauce-to-noodle balance. Sprinkle in any or all the herbs and, if you like, the nutritional yeast. It adds body, flavor, and oomph. Toss to combine and season generously with sea salt and a good grinding of fresh pepper.

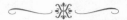

GENTLE NUDGE *the* NINTH:
GET CAUGHT UP *in the* RAPTURE

Vegetables get their name from the Latin *vegetare*, which means "to enliven." It's life force, chi, all that stuff. Processed food, on the other hand, must have its origins in the word *zombie*. So eat a vegetable — a fresh vegetable. It can change your life. Changed mine.

My mother used to be into Atkins (don't get me started); my father is vegphobic. Fresh green vegetables weren't part of my childhood. Vegetables came in a frozen brick — it was a benighted era; we knew no better. They were something relegated. An afterthought. To this day, my father will manage to choke down a fresh asparagus tip then give up and say the hell with it.

My childhood involved eating a fair amount of bad (that is to say, frozen) broccoli. And yet, in one of those mysteries of life, I grew to love vegetables, all of them, starting with broccoli, my first vegetable love. Like all true loves, it has endured. I didn't go looking for broccoli but stumbled upon it, where it was waiting for me all along.

My sophomore year of college, I was home on summer break, helping to make dinner. I'd steamed a head of fresh broccoli, intending, as was family tradition, to bury it under buttered bread crumbs — the better to disguise it. I was separating the florets with my fingers when I absentmindedly popped one in my mouth. Everything stopped.

I surrendered to the taste, vegetal yet sweet, and to the texture, firm to the bite yet yielding. I fell upon the broccoli, unbuttered, uncrumbed, unadorned, like a woman starving. I could all but feel its phytonutrients working their magic on me, busting through bad college food and worse college habits. I'd been a vegetarian for years, but in that instant, I became something more — a broccoli believer, my life forever changed, redeemed, hallelujah.

Vegetable rapture can happen to you, too. But you've got to engage with the process. Start by eating a fresh vegetable.

Broccoli with Lemon and Mint (Broccoli for Beginners)

Serves 4

1 head broccoli
1 bunch fresh mint
1 lemon, halved
Olive oil for drizzling
Sea salt for sprinkling

Take one lovely green head of broccoli. Rinse off the invisible nasties. Cut into florets, leaving on as much stem as you can stand. That's where the phytonutrients are. Tossing out the broccoli stem wastes resources and cheats you out of the best nutritional bits. Steamed, the woody stems turn tender and kind of great tasting — like asparagus. Chop them into bits and you've got bonus broccoli.

Do you want to be plunged into boiling water? Neither does broccoli. Steaming preserves the nutrients in produce, so invest in a covered steamer or double boiler. Place the broccoli — florets and chopped stems — in the top pot, the one with the holes at the bottom. Fill the pot below halfway with water. Bring the water to a boil over high heat. Cover and steam for 7 minutes, then peek inside and check on your broccoli's progress. It should smell vegetal and rich and be glowing and green. You want stems that snap, not bend. Give it another minute or two, if needed, then rinse in cold water or toss a handful of ice into the steamer. Like other vegetables, broccoli retains heat and will continue cooking until you bring down its temperature.

Stop to admire. You have just steamed fresh broccoli and it is beautiful. Do a little broccoli dance.

Take the naked broccoli florets and the chopped stems, and throw them in a bowl. Take a few handfuls of fragrant mint, chop or tear into bits, and throw it in too. Squeeze the juice of 1 lemon over the broccoli and drizzle it with olive oil. Toss. Sprinkle with sea salt. Eat as a salad, as a side dish, or like it's popcorn.

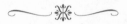

Let your whim and the season guide you. Because whatever vegetable you choose will offer you something fabulous, be it cold-friendly kale in the winter, with off-the-charts amounts of antioxidants, calcium, iron, and vitamin C, or the first tender peas of spring — vitamin K, folate, zinc! That's why Hippocrates said, "Let food be thy medicine and medicine be thy food."

Still more taken by the big, the blingy? More by the Kardashian sisters than you are by kale? Behold the kale chip.

All you need are three ingredients and ten minutes to transform the leafy green you've been avoiding into addictive finger food.

Kale Chips

Change up the flavor by mixing the sea salt with a pinch of cumin, red pepper flakes, curry powder, thyme, or any dried herb or spice you like.

Serves 4

1 bunch kale
2 teaspoons olive oil
Sea salt for sprinkling

Preheat the oven to 300°F.

Wash the kale leaves and blot dry. Tear or cut the leaves free of the stems. (Reserve the stems for vegetable broth.) Tear the leaves into generous-size chips, keeping in mind that the chips will shrink during baking. Place the kale pieces on a large baking sheet. Drizzle with olive oil and toss until the leaves are evenly coated with the oil. Sprinkle with sea salt.

Bake in the oven for 10 minutes. The kale will shrink down and turn magically crispy.

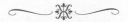

FEEDING *the* HUNGRY GHOST

Our first year in Tokyo, Benjamin and I discovered Japan has street festivals every weekend all spring and summer long — cherry blossom festival, plum festival, festivals all around town, with the people in each prefecture parading their own shrine through the neighborhood. They all seem to feature happy crowds and street vendors selling grilled squid on a stick. We'd know we were closing on the festival location when we'd get that squiddy whiff of burned tires.

One summer evening, we were out walking and stumbled onto an event we hadn't known about. It had squid, but it felt different. It felt hushed, as though everyone was holding their breath.

Women in their crisp *yukata* (cotton summer kimonos) and men in dark suits and ties clustered by the banks of the winding Sumida River in the fading light of day. They lit candles and set them afloat in little paper boats. Then they would bow and release them out on the water. When darkness fell, the sky was lit with fireworks, what the Japanese call *hanabi* — "fire flowers." But I kept turning back to look at the glow of the candles in their boats, floating out and away.

The next day, the proprietress of the noodle shop downstairs explained this was the week of Obon, when the dead return to visit their living families. The families gather, pray for them, do a little dance, place fruits and vegetables on the family altar, tidy up the graves of the dead, then send them off in the candle ceremony we'd witnessed.

One of the things I like best about human beings is our ability to make a party out of anything. The dead are busting loose? Outstanding. Let's dance, let's make them feel welcome, let's cook. What's their favorite thing to eat, besides squid on a stick? Japan's *other* street food — donburi.

Donburi means something served over rice — usually eggs. It's easy, popular; it's Japanese comfort food. I've enriched it by adding vegetables. And losing the egg. It's still excellent.

Vegetable Donburi

Serves 2

2 cups water
1 cup rice (white is traditional, brown is more healthful)
1 cup Stone Soup (see page 84) or other vegetable broth
¼ cup sake or sherry
1 tablespoon white miso paste
1 tablespoon soy sauce
2 teaspoons sesame oil (optional)
2 cups broccoli florets
2 carrots, chopped
1 teaspoon minced fresh ginger
2 cloves garlic, minced
8 ounces mushrooms, sliced
4 scallions, chopped

In a medium saucepan, bring the water to a boil over high heat. Add the rice, cover, and reduce the heat to low. Simmer until all the liquid is absorbed and the rice is tender, about 30 minutes for white rice, 40 minutes for brown rice. Remove from the heat, with the saucepan covered to keep the rice warm.

In another medium saucepan, bring the broth to a boil over high heat. Add the sake, miso paste, soy sauce, and sesame oil (if using). Stir together until smooth. Add the broccoli, carrots, ginger, and garlic and cook for 2 minutes, or until the vegetables soften. Add the mushrooms and scallions and cook, giving the vegetables a brisk, light stir, until the mushrooms turn dark, soft, and juicy and all the vegetables are heated through, a few minutes more.

Divide the cooked rice into two bowls. Gently spoon the vegetables and their sauce on top.

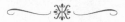

In Hong Kong, Benjamin and I discovered Yu Lan, the Hungry Ghost Festival, much as we had come upon Obon in Tokyo — by accident. We were on summer holiday, walking along Cat Street, with its dazzle of antique and apothecary shops, the street vendors holding up their wares. They called out in English and Cantonese, their shouts ringing together like music. Amid the bustle of vendors, I spied a woman with a cooler full of ice. She was selling fresh lychees. There may be some for whom grilled squid on a stick sates a deep and urgent craving, but for me, it's chilled lychees on a gloriously hot afternoon. We bought a bag and went on our way, peeling the fruit, popping the cold sweetness into each other's mouths. We had no destination in mind, no schedule to keep; the day was its own reward.

We came to a temple surrounded by a fug of incense. Through the high open doors, we saw people bowing and praying as if their lives depended on it.

In theory, China's Yu Lan is similar to Japan's Obon. It's an honoring of the dead, but it translates into something edgier. In China, hungry ghosts are seriously hungry, depicted with teeny little mouths, narrow, reedy necks, and big, empty bellies that can never get enough.

Oh, they might venture back to their living kin for a reunion, but they're more likely to hang out in the water, waiting till you take a refreshing swim. Then they'll pull you down and under. They're dead, depleted, ravenous, and in a bad mood.

Like Obon, Yu Lan involves prayers and altars and food offerings, but the consumables are more likely to be a pack of smokes and a bottle of scotch. It's not healthy, but what does it matter? They're offerings for people already dead. Booze and ciggies are what they want — or what we think they want — and it's better they're appeased. Or else.

Go ahead, blame the dead. They're not corporeally here to defend themselves. I think we're more often the ones who want more, more, more. Even better, we want you to have less.

Some of the seven deadly sins are fun — lust comes to mind. Gluttony, sloth, and pride also have their appeal. Of all of them, I get plagued by envy, your real downer sin. I can tell you, too much wanting gets in the way of living, the way too much salt ruins the dish, scours your taste buds, and makes it so you can enjoy none of it. And it's exhausting. Bad enough to be that way when I'm alive; I'm not going through it when I'm dead.

A little desire, a little appetite, is sexy. Even in a ghost. It means you're open to receiving the world's pleasures. The question is, what are you hungry for? If you knew almost ten billion animals are killed every year for food, would you really want seconds on the barbecue?

We're hungry for more than dinner. I am, anyway. There's not a bunch of kale or head of broccoli or loaf of zucchini bread big enough to fill the ache, the hole, the hunger to be more, to be better.

Often — mostly late at night — my insecurities come out and dance. They've got the moves; they've got the looks. Meanwhile, I'm lying there awake and fat and old and stupid and ugly. This is what my insecurities tell me, anyway. While they're dancing. Through perfectly lipsticked lips, they remind me I'm not Deepak Chopra. Or today's Food Network star. Or Lady Gaga (though they know I would never, ever do her meat-dress thing). Or you.

When necessary, I visualize rushing out on that dance floor

and tripping them. Then I rip off their false eyelashes and hair extensions. When I can prize my grip off my obsession du soir, the thing I lack, that I must have or die, I am — human paradox — less hungry for it. It is a matter of breathing through the crazies.

I strive for *enoughness*, feeling complete with what I have and who I am. It is not all about me. Lady Gaga probably has bad days, too. Perhaps another word for this is *perspective*.

The next recipe is one of those Zen, less-is-more kinds of things, perfect for when your inner hungry ghost is being particularly pesky. It requires many vegetables and a bit of prep. Embrace the process; it's there to get you out of your own head. It's a simplified version of Buddha's Delight, the traditional mild and meatless monk's stew that brings good health and good fortune. Its selling point isn't spice, but a symphony of textures. It delighted an enlightened guy like Buddha. May it work for you, too.

Hungry Ghost Mood Modifier

Shirataki are low-calorie, gluten-free noodles made from sweet potato, with an interesting chew. They require no cooking, come packed in water, and can have an off-putting smell when you open the bag. Don't be afraid; just rinse them well. Find shirataki, along with rice vinegar and sesame oil, at most Asian markets and natural food stores.

Serves 2

2 teaspoons canola or peanut oil
1 clove garlic, minced

1 thumb-size piece fresh ginger, peeled and cut into
   matchsticks
2 scallions, chopped
1 carrot, cut into matchsticks
1 stalk celery, chopped
1 red bell pepper, cut into matchsticks
1 cup shredded cabbage
4 ounces firm tofu, cut into bite-size cubes
2 tablespoons soy sauce
1 tablespoon Asian rice vinegar
1 teaspoon agave nectar or honey
1 teaspoon sesame oil
One 8-ounce package shirataki, rinsed well and drained

In a large skillet, heat the oil over medium-high heat. Add the garlic, ginger, and scallions. Cook, stirring occasionally, until the vegetables are fragrant and softened, about 2 minutes.

Add the carrot, celery, and red bell pepper. Cooking, stirring occasionally, until they become tender, 2 to 3 minutes more.

Add the cabbage and tofu. Cook, stirring occasionally to prevent the vegetables and tofu from sticking to the bottom of the pan. Cabbage wilts quickly, so this will only take 3 to 5 minutes.

In a small bowl, whisk together the soy sauce, rice vinegar, agave nectar, and sesame oil. Pour the mixture over the vegetables and tofu, and stir gently until evenly coated.

Add the shirataki and toss to combine. Cook, giving a gentle stir, until the sauce is mostly absorbed and the shirataki is heated through, a few minutes more.

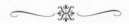

Maybe ghosts really do spend their days directing us, in which case they're as busy in the next life as in this one. No wonder some of them get cranky. Or maybe the haunting is of our own making — regret or anger over the things we did and didn't do, longing for what was, pain over what we want that can never be again. In either case, it is unfinished business.

It helps us to honor and commemorate the dead. It makes it easier for us. And who knows? Maybe it helps them, too. Who doesn't like being remembered and showered with presents? But we have no proof a bottle of scotch or a handful of lychees tastes as good to a spirit as it does when you still have a physical self. Another thing being alive has going for it — there's still time to buff over the rough spots in our personalities. There's still time to make it right.

I don't know what the dead need, but the living need at least two Hungry Ghost Festivals. The frantic approach of throwing booze at our ancestors in the hopes they'll leave us alone reflects the way things are when you scrape below the surface — it's all our raw feelings, our fears, our own hungry ghosts. The demure family get-together, complete with candles and squid, reflects a desire to draw around us those we love, now while we are still living, when we can clank around in our clever bag of bones, engaging with all our senses, from scotch's medicinal tang and smoky notes to the spiced sweetness of lychees.

So do it now. Feed yourself and those you love. Or even those you like. It is summer, the harvest is bountiful, and we are alive.

GENTLE NUDGE *the* TENTH: BALANCING ACT

Sitting on my desk is a statuette of Ganesh, the Hindu elephant-headed god, god of the harvest and remover of obstacles. In many representations, Ganesh is seated, looking benign and slightly pleased with the universe — or himself. He is the god of success, after all. My Ganesh is dancing. Or at least poised to dance. He is balanced on one foot, the other leg raised and bent, his arms extended in graceful waves, the position belly dancers call serpentine.

I'm a belly-dance dropout, but I, too, can balance on one foot. I often do this when on the phone or waiting in line at the bank or post office — it's an easy way to multitask, it kills the time, it works the abs. I can balance when I'm still, but we're not still, are we? We're always moving.

Even when we're at rest, our brains are active. Sometimes, they're just willful. My brain regularly wakes from a semisound sleep around three in the morning and takes the rest of me hostage, treating me to a double feature of stupid things I've done wrong during the day and things I'm behind on and may never get to.

This does not encourage a return to sleep. It encourages hours of unproductive worry. I can get myself crazy and out of balance by lying absolutely still. It's a talent I'm not especially proud of.

Balance is something we crave with our whole being. Balance does not mean blandness; it means stability. It is like the Tao symbol of yin and yang, two equal parts, light and dark, female and male, curled into each other to make a perfect circle, a completeness.

Perfect and complete are hard to keep up. We are made up of opposites, but when one side exerts more force than the other, we get knocked down — by life, by stress, by the nasty flu making the rounds in the office. We crave balance, but we're not good at it. We work too hard at the expense of the relationships that sustain us — our families, our communities, ourselves. We're running on empty, and we're hungry, depleted. But we don't stop; we keep bouncing and banging from extreme to extreme, from starving to stuffing our faces. Again and again. Bad use of energy. And doesn't it seem extreme and just the littlest bit, um, insane? The Hopi have a word for it — *koyaanisqatsi*. It means "crazy life." It means "life out of balance." Philip Glass composed a stirring musical score by that name. It is in turns frenetic and sonorous and moody and ominous. It is not the sound track you want for your life.

Even a hurricane, that convection of fury, has a center point of stillness. And that's the trick. Finding balance means slowing down, finding that moment of stillness in the midst of the dance, that one thing we think we're far too busy to do. I am sorry to say you cannot achieve balance with a pill or a Wii. But you can do it yourself. Meditate.

Meditation reminds us we are each a bright glow of energy but a small part of a very large world. It increases mindfulness. It refreshes the spirit and body. It's proven to lower blood pressure and increase focus. And it's hard.

What I once called meditating meant sitting with every muscle clenched, my face scrunched with anxiety, because the great cosmic answers were not coming to me. This is not what meditation is. It's about allowing yourself to be, to accept who and where you are in the world right now.

I have to think of meditation as a marathon run by sitting absolutely still. It takes training, and it takes patience. On the upside, you don't need any expensive gear. I have yet to get the promised runner's high. Maybe next time.

Sitting silently with myself makes my brain go berserk with a million useless thoughts. I need to make some calls. Isn't that the phone ringing now? My left leg is all pins and needles. It's going to sleep. Or else it's something dire. Maybe I'm having an aneurysm. How can you tell? Must do a Google search. Must check my email, or I will die. Breathe. Jesus, I'm really in the zone now. Hours must have gone by. I open my left eye and check the clock. Actual time elapsed — forty-nine seconds.

The world will wait. It's patient. I return to following my breathing, to clearing my brain. My brain should have its own yard sale — no! Don't think yard sale. Don't think. Just be. Just breathe.

You've got to be better at this than I am. Block out fifteen minutes for yourself. No phone calls, no interruptions. Find a restful place. Sit comfortably, quietly, your feet on the floor. Your chair, your couch will support you, the soles of your feet connect you to the energy of the whole benevolent planet. You're being looked after, so let go. Close your eyes. Open your mind and your heart. Focus on your breath, the gentle rhythm of it, the rise and fall of your chest. It's elegant, and you do it all the time without even appreciating it. Clever you. So while you're sitting there, just send your body a message. Tell it thank you.

You do not have to do this forever. Just for now. Give yourself permission to do what we're always saying we need to do — be here now.

While you're in this receptive, meditative state, contemplate what you need in order to be balanced, what you need to thrive. Think about how you live and what you eat and what you can tweak to nourish your excellent body and luminous soul.

We can't be conscious of the seasons of the earth until we are conscious of our own seasons. We can't be stewards of the land when we're not able to take care of ourselves. Meditation gives you a break from your busy, busy day so you can listen to yourself. What are you saying? You may not get an instant answer. Breathe. Relax. In time, it will become clear.

In the meantime, here you are. You are enough, you are

plenty. Because if you want to look at the larger picture (and I always do), harvest means more than what you pull out of the field. It is the reward you reap for effort expended; it is the sum of who you are right now. And you are a lavish harvest.

You wouldn't think meditating takes energy — you're just sitting there — but it does. And you want to fuel yourself properly. A bowl of oats provides a bowl of low-glycemic, heart-supporting, whole grain goodness that stops hunger in its tracks and can help you find focus. If all you know is instant, it is time to branch out and try the pebbly wonder of steel-cut oats. They require a longer cooking time but provide ample reward by way of satiety and a full, nutty flavor.

I have added goji berries, the wonder berry of the moment. They are another ancient gift we're just discovering. People say gojis boost circulation, immunity, and liver function. What people don't tell you is gojis are slightly sour and chewy. When cooked in with the oats, though, they soften in flavor and texture and become entirely more agreeable.

Steel-Cut Oats with Goji Berries

Now is a good time to get into that meditative, serene state. Steel-cut oats are not your basic rolled oats. They're cut crosswise, so they're pebbly, not flaky, and have oaten oomph. They also require twice as much water and twice as much time to cook. But they are delicious, filling, and fabulous for you.

Enjoy topped with flaxseeds, hemp seeds, chia seeds, nuts, any manner of berries or chopped fruit, dried or fresh, a lavish sprinkle of cinnamon, a drizzle of maple syrup, whatever pleases you. I know someone who enjoys soy sauce on his oatmeal, but he's a genius and can get away with it.

Serves 2 (or Ganesh all by himself)

2 cups water
½ cup steel-cut oats
2 tablespoons dried goji berries
1 teaspoon ground cinnamon
1 teaspoon agave nectar or maple syrup

In a medium saucepan, bring the water to a boil over high heat. Add the oats and goji berries and cook, stirring occasionally, until the oats thicken, a few minutes.

Reduce the heat to low and cook, uncovered and stirring occasionally, until the oats and water magically coalesce to optimal creaminess, 20 to 30 minutes.

Stir in the cinnamon and agave nectar, then enjoy as is or lavish with toppings to your heart's delight.

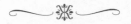

Chapter

4 *the* COMPOST

Anyone can tell it's autumn when the temperature drops and the leaves change color. In South Florida, a place not otherwise known for subtlety, the change in seasons is so slight, newcomers don't even notice. You have to live here awhile to be awake to the way the light shifts, from bright and bleached-out to a softer sunshine that bathes everything in gold. The humidity lifts, and with it, our hearts.

Snow is for other people. From Key Biscayne to the Everglades, my beloved waterbirds are nesting — brown pelicans flying above in phalanx; snowy egrets rocking their vampy breeding plumage; plump, placid purple gallinules that look like bath-time rubber ducks dressed up with jewellike iridescent feathers.

Now is our planting season, a time of growth and nurturing. Yet at the same time that I'm putting in my kale, arugula, chard, peppers, radishes, and tomatoes, I can also sense the presence of ghosts.

Even in Miami, where October heat and humidity can turn

a fierce jack-o'-lantern into a pile of pumpkin puree overnight, something is in the air. We shift back to standard time, and by early evening, the sky is black, as though the sun had decided to call it quits forever and it's the end of the universe as we know it.

You can see how this might weird people out.

Before Halloween was an excuse to eat candy and a ghost meant a costume made of a bedsheet with two holes cut out for eyes, the ancient Celts believed late autumn was the time of the dead, when they came back to earth because they hadn't gotten to cross everything off their to-do list. The Celts marked the time with feasting and celebration to honor the dead. They hoped if they acted nice, the dead would feel mollified and go back where they came from. Druids did the same thing but added orgies.

By the eighth century, the Catholic Church had grown in influence; the church said, enough of this orgy business, cleaned up the sex, and designated November 1 as All Saints' Day. But you know, the people like their sex and wildness, so the church had to add All Souls' Day on November 2. People didn't get to have sex, at least not church-sanctioned sex, but they could have bonfires and dress up in funky gear.

Benjamin and I observe a cleaned-up, modern Halloween. We take our young niece Nikki to pick out a pumpkin from the Boys Club sale, then bring her back to our house to carve it. This tradition dates back not to the Celts, but to my girlhood. I did it — and still do it — with my father. We've been doing it for decades, and yet our carving skills have scarcely improved. Each year, our jack-o'-lantern features triangle eyes and nose and an orthodontist's dream of a snaggletoothed smile.

On Halloween, we light our jack-o'-lantern and dispense candy to adorable trick-or-treaters, me doing it with a fair amount of guilt for feeding them junk. On the other hand, I'm not going to be the neighborhood mean, crazy lady doling out apples or homemade flaxseed bonbons. I tried giving out handfuls of pennies one year, shining them up with lemon juice and salt, pretty, pretty. Never again. No wonder we're left off any orgy A-lists. Things, though, are far from tame.

Pumpkin, Poblano, and Spinach Tacos

Seasonal produce delivers heat, sweet, and nourishment with vitamins A, B, and C, calcium, iron, potassium, and oh, I could keep going. Jack-o'-lanterns, though tempting to use (because we hate to waste, don't we?), go mushy and bland when cooked. Choose a more flavorful variety like cheese pumpkin or sugar pumpkin for this southwestern-inspired meal.

Epazote, a traditional Mexican herb, has a grassy, savory flavor and has been used as a stomach soother. It also goes by wormseed and the more appealing name Jesuit's tea.

Serves 6 to 8

4 poblano peppers
One 2-pound pumpkin, cut into bite-size cubes
2 tablespoons olive oil
Sea salt and freshly ground pepper
1 good-size onion, chopped
2 cloves garlic, chopped
Pinch dried epazote, or pinch dried oregano and pinch
   dried thyme
Leaves from 1 sprig fresh sage, chopped
4 big handfuls spinach
6 to 10 multigrain or corn tortillas
Toasted pepitas (pumpkin seeds) for garnish (optional)

Shredded vegan cheese for garnish (optional)

Hot sauce for garnish (optional)

Place one rack in the uppermost position of the oven and another rack in the middle position. Preheat the broiler. Place the poblanos on a baking sheet on the top rack and broil until blackened on both sides, 8 to 10 minutes per side.

Remove the poblanos from the oven and immediately wrap them in a kitchen towel or seal them in a paper bag. Let the poblanos sweat for at least 20 minutes. When they're cool enough to handle, slip off the blistered skins. Remove the seeds and cut the peppers into bite-size strips. (The roasted peppers can be wrapped and stored in the refrigerator for a day.)

Turn off the broiler and set the oven to 425°F.

Spread the pumpkin cubes on a rimmed baking sheet. Drizzle with 1 tablespoon of the olive oil, and season with salt and pepper. Roast on the middle rack until light brown and tender, about 30 minutes, giving the vegetables an occasional flip or stir so they roast evenly.

Meanwhile, in a large skillet, heat the remaining 1 tablespoon olive oil over medium-high heat. Add the onion and garlic. Cook, stirring occasionally, until the onion is softened and golden, about 8 minutes. Add the epazote, poblano strips, and sage.

Reduce the heat to medium. Add the roasted pumpkin and the spinach, a handful at a time, and cook until the spinach just wilts and the pumpkin and poblanos are heated through, 5 to 7 minutes. Taste and season with salt and pepper

To warm the tortillas, wrap in a kitchen towel and steam in a double boiler for a minute or two, or wrap in aluminum foil and place in a 300°F oven for a minute or two.

Mound the filling onto tortillas. Top the tacos with toasted pepitas, shredded vegan cheese, and perhaps a splash of hot sauce, and enjoy.

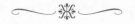

I've barely pitched the putrefied Halloween pumpkin into our compost bin when bang, it's time to do the big cleanup and cook for Thanksgiving. Then comes the wave of holiday parties, and it's a quick skid to Christmas, Hanukkah, New Year's Eve, all coming at you so fast, you don't even have time to take the leaves out of the dining-room table. Where did the past few months go? Where did the year go?

We see the end of the calendar, have the sense that time is running out, and start to feel the wee-est bit desperate. Silly us. Time is a human construct. For the planet, winter is just another cycle, a gearing down, a storing up.

On the surface, the world may show itself as forbidding gray skies, barren trees, snow-covered fields or slush-crusted streets, and other End of Days indicators. Really, the party's just starting.

You know how a good night's sleep smoothes out your forehead and your spirits, and makes it possible for you to keep on with a smile? That's how the earth feels, too. A winter's nap perks up the planet. Your body temperature drops when you sleep. Earth's does, too. But deep within, there's still sweetness and warmth and growth. This is the time for filling, nourishing root vegetables, like beets, carrots, and sweet potatoes. They laugh at cold temperatures and keep for months in your larder. Note their tonality, in the red-to-orange scheme of things — the colors we associate with heat. You could almost think there was some grand design behind it.

With the colder, shorter days of winter, we, too, seek sweetness and warmth deep within ourselves, the promise of renewal. Think of it as a spa experience for your soul — a spiritual sloughing off, a mystical exfoliation.

There's a reason the evergreen is a Christmas symbol. It's green even in the heart of winter, reminding us this is a season of regeneration. For all of us. The liturgical calendar begins not in the springtime with obvious new life and pretty green leaves, but in December. Now is the season of Advent, of contemplation and togetherness, of readying, of preparing to party, should the Savior come, of being cheerful and carrying on if he gets hung up in traffic or if it doesn't happen at all. We are ready to begin.

In Judaism, winter is the time of Simchat Torah. We have read through the entire Torah, the sacred Hebrew scroll, over the course of the year. We have reached the end. And yet not the end. We get to end and begin again, at the beginning.

The planet teaches us things do not end, or if they do, these endings are never as neat or dramatic as we humans make them seem at the time. I'm glad. I hate good-byes.

We can't erase the past. We need the past. We couldn't have reached this shiny, new moment without it — even Janus, the god of beginnings, knows that.

January is named for Janus. You can tell him from all the other gods because he's the one with two heads, one looking forward into the future and the other facing backward, to gaze into the past. You are not who you were ten years ago or even ten months ago. Every year, every season, lays the groundwork for what is to come. Think of time as metaphoric compost, primordial muck, the broken-down organic matter creating the perfect environment in which to grow, to begin again.

Life is messy. Just working on an art project with your kid will teach you that. It'll turn your dining-room table into a Jackson Pollock of glue-gun dribbles that, like Lady Macbeth's bloodstained hands, will never come clean. But your child doesn't see that; he sees a priceless work of art he created. You want to crap on that? Look, he has the rest of his life to wallow in guilt and disappointment. You helped bring a masterpiece to fruition. You have prepared the soil, you have created a fertile, sacred space. Birth comes from decay. Kinda odd, but there you go.

WILDCAT SCATTER

If you live long enough, someone you love is going to die. What happens then, whether the dead enter the realm of heaven, receive divine enlightenment, come back as a ghost or a cow or compost, is unknown to those of us still living. What happens to us, though, is no mystery at all. Losing someone you love hurts like hell.

This is when formal religions should step it up, plugging in faith and support. In the West, your bigger religions often provide a guidebook — when you feel this way, read or say or do that. This isn't always far enough, to judge by the uptick in secular ceremonies, a DIY approach to death, as it were.

You want more than words; you want a ritual, one that says hey, world, pay attention — we've lost one of the great ones. You want a ceremony that's meaningful, not just to you, but to the person you're honoring. So you do something like spread your beloved's ashes somewhere that mattered, somewhere that provided joy. And if it means doing so without getting approval, you will do it anyway. Furtively. Under cover of darkness. With a backup plan in case it all goes wrong, and armed with a bottle of the dearly departed's favorite brand of booze for communion and comfort. This is known in the funerary biz as wildcat scatter.

A large and solid person in life becomes light after cremation. Spreading the ashes ("cremains" — another funerary term) feels rather like spreading organic fertilizer, which, in a sense, it is. But nature has its limits. Even the most fertile soil won't grow the person you lost back to life. There's no way to bring back the dead.

Unless it is memory. Memory is its own sort of wildcat scatter. Call them ghosts, call them memories of the dead, they surround me, infuse me. I believe in ghosts. John Milton did, too. Or at least he wrote about it convincingly enough in *Paradise Lost*: "Millions of spiritual creatures walk the Earth / Unseen, both when we wake, and when we sleep."

I feel their presence as a tender ache in my heart, a whisper in my ear, the sizzle of something in a pan, a whiff of Marcella's L'Air du Temps or the tang of the gin my father-in-law loved, a poke in the ribs, a desire to laugh and cry at once that isn't PMS. I do not hear voices telling me to fight for France, but sometimes, especially toward the end of the year, I'll hear, "I could go for a little something before lunch," and I'll smile, remembering Patrick, my first boss, who loved coffee and cookies and, oddly enough, me.

Almond Cookies

Patrick and I agreed life is hard enough without hard cookies. These tender treats are Chinese in origin, but untraditional, being lardless.

Makes 2 dozen cookies

½ cup (1 stick) vegan margarine, such as Earth Balance, softened
1 tablespoon almond butter
⅔ cup evaporated cane sugar

2 teaspoons amaretto
⅔ cup almond flour
⅔ cup unbleached all-purpose flour
1 teaspoon aluminum-free baking powder
A neutral oil like canola for the baking sheet
24 blanched almonds*

In a large bowl, use a mixing spoon to cream together the vegan margarine, almond butter, and sugar. Stir together for a few minutes, until the mixture is light and fluffy. Mix in the amaretto and almond flour until just combined.

In another large bowl, sift together the all-purpose flour and baking powder. Add the flour mixture to the butter-sugar mixture and stir until just combined. The dough will be slightly sticky.

Turn out the dough onto a lightly floured surface and shape it into a log about 12 inches long and 1½ inches in diameter. Wrap well in aluminum foil and refrigerate at least 2 hours or up to overnight.

When ready to bake, preheat the oven to 350°F. Lightly oil a rimmed baking sheet.

Unwrap the dough and slice into ½-inch-thick rounds. Place the dough rounds, 2 inches apart, on the prepared baking sheet. Gently press a blanched almond into the center of each cookie. Bake until the cookies are just turning golden, 10 to 12 minutes.

Remove from the oven and let cool. The cookies are quite tender indeed fresh from the oven, but they firm up as they cool.

Store in an airtight container for several days.

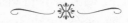

---

* To blanch almonds, pour whole raw almonds into a small heatproof bowl. Cover with boiling water and let sit for 15 minutes. Drain. The almond skins will slip off easily, leaving you perfect, pale nut kernels.

You can also work a different kind of magic with this version, which whispers of the Middle East.

Variation: Orange Blossom Cookies

Grate in 1 teaspoon orange zest
Substitute 1 teaspoon orange-flower water* for the
     2 teaspoons amaretto
Increase the unbleached all-purpose flour to ¾ cup
Substitute pine nuts for the almonds

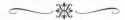

I met Patrick when I was seventeen and somehow got hired as media-relations assistant for a local arts festival. My first day, he shambled in late, a black-and-white cookie as big as Manhattan sticking out of his mouth, a Styrofoam cup of coffee in his hand. He wore a rumpled madras plaid shirt not quite tucked into his khakis. I was inexperienced but not naive. I could tell this guy was not standard issue.

Patrick's disordered style belied his superpowers. He could take the measure of a situation and make the best of it. In our many cookie-and-coffee klatches, he explained our job was not about creating beautiful content with artistic vision, but about placating rude people, defusing ticketing disasters, and doing damage control when a famous playwright shows up drunk, knocks over a tray of canapés, and does something unspeakable to the hostess.

---

* Orange-flower water is available in Middle Eastern and gourmet markets.

Patrick was indispensable. To everyone. He would walk into a crowded room, and even with a celeb or two in the mix, he was the one everyone was glad to see.

At the end of summer, the festival ended seriously in the red, and the organizers pulled the plug on ever having another. I went back to college for my sophomore year, now skilled in the ways of appeasing the entitled, tracking down AWOL artists, and finagling free drinks. The end.

Except Patrick wouldn't let it be. He called every week, even after he moved to New York with his new partner, Marc. They showed up in Miami around Christmas. We took holidays together. Here's a picture of us at a tatty Miami attraction, with nasty-clawed macaws sitting on our heads. They're heavier than you'd think. Here's another picture of us swimming laps in a neighbor's hot tub. And here's me in bridal getup, flanked by my gorgeous new husband on one side and Patrick and Marc on the other. Patrick is feeding me wedding cake — carrot, really good — tuxedo shirttail already hanging out of his pants. Marc is giving me sips of champagne; we're all laughing at the great joke of life. It's a wonderful, joyful image; but more than that, it says to the world, we're not just husband and wife — we're Benjamin and Ellen and Patrick and Marc, and that's the way it was and would always be forever.

It should have been. You may sense where I'm going with this.

Patrick got a cold. It lasted a long time. He had pneumonia, edema, a bunch of miseries that were not going away and did not add up to a common cold. He got hepatitis — the wrong kind. Despite our physical distance and my busy life, I had to face the facts — my friend was dying.

Marc called one December day. "It's going to be soon," he said. "Patrick wants you to be here."

All my life I'd agonized over everything. But this was very clear. I booked a flight, baked a batch of almond cookies, and flew out the next day, taking a cab straight from the airport to the hospital. It was midwinter; the hospital was dreary and gray and encrusted with gray ice.

Patrick's room, though, was stifling hot and full of people. It was like all the cocktail parties we'd attended (or crashed), except for one thing — in bed was someone who was my friend and yet not my friend. With his red hair and beard and the hammy thighs he worried about, my Patrick looked like a fun Vincent Van Gogh who ate well and had both his ears. This guy was wasted, emaciated, hooked up to every kind of tube. His eyes and skin were the color of French's mustard. He was never going to eat cookies again, ever.

I could feel my tears start; but he hated that, so I hugged him. He felt like kindling. He said, "You feel good." I said I'd just had this spa treatment where they sanded my ass.

"Lemme feel." Whatever he had become, he was still Patrick.

I undid my jeans and slipped his hand in — gently, because it was bony and rigged to things doing I had no idea what.

The party didn't last long; it was clear people didn't want to stick around. It wasn't just because I'd presented my backside.

So it was just Patrick and Marc and me and an uneaten box of cookies. Sometimes we'd chat, sometimes we fell silent. A lot of the time, Patrick moaned. Over the next days, I got good at untwisting his tubes and swabbing his mouth with a glycerin stick. Sometimes I'd put his hand on my ass, and he'd almost smile.

One morning, he began convulsing. He yanked at his tubes and thrashed and shouted. He didn't know who we were; but he looked at me, and in his eyes, yellowed with jaundice, I saw anger, frustration, and horror, a sense of, how could we let this happen?

"Morphine reaction," the doctor said. "It's normal." Not for me. I went down the hall, turned to the wall, held up my cell phone without turning it on and said, "I can't do this, I can't do this, I can't do this."

Then I took a breath. Patrick didn't want to do this, either. But he didn't have a choice. So I put my phone away and went back and stayed with him. Sometimes the only thing you can do is witness, try to bear another's pain. It is times like these that faith must come in handy, like a pair of jumper cables. Me, I felt hobbled by helplessness.

A nurse gave Patrick an injection and he finally calmed and grew still. Marc left to take a break, and I, exhausted, curled up in bed with my friend and took a nap.

That evening, Marc and I sat in Patrick's room, talking quietly while he slept, guarding him, listening to the rasp of his breath. Then we both looked at Patrick at the same moment and realized — he was gone. It felt very like he had left the room. I saw a silver mist, like a sprinkling of snow or powdered sugar, hovering above him just a moment, then it was gone. It is pretty and pleasing to think it was Patrick's spirit. More likely it was lack of sleep on my part.

Marcella had died by then. And Aaron. But you're not supposed to die when you're in your thirties. You're not supposed to die when you're Patrick.

In grief, your carefully constructed life crashes and falls away, leaving you exposed, flayed, raw, helpless as a newborn. Daily life becomes a matrix of impossibilities, starting with getting out of bed in the morning. You develop sleep alternatives or new ways of grooming. That they might not be successful is beside the point.

At other times, grief feels like a bone lodged in the throat, a calcification of the heart. The bits of you that ought to be open are obstructed. The pain of loss dulls your senses, creates a force field around your body, encases you in ice, makes you impervious to the world around you, and especially impervious to its pleasures. You shut down.

Grief is a necessary pain. That means there's no way around it — try to bury it now, and it'll come back and tsunami you later. But when you're grieving, the world grants you a little slack. You have license to be weird. In fact, you need to be. It's the only way you're going to get through it. Think of it as a healthy madness.

People you know and people you don't will say or do things intended to comfort. Not all of them will help, like someone telling you it's for the best. I do not recommend responding, as I did, "Oh, really? And when did you become God?"

People will tell you how it was when their friend/lover/spouse/parent/pet died. And for every twenty people, one will say something that will make you blink, that will resonate and make you ask, "It was like that for you, too?" Because we all grieve, in our own ways and our own time. No one gets out of it.

In the wake of death, people bring food. The precedent is as old as humankind and initially was about feeding not the living, but the dead. The Celts believed the journey from life to death was hard work, requiring fortification by way of eats — or what they called *lón báis* (death sustenance). It didn't take long for folks to realize those left behind to mourn weren't having a day at the beach, either. And we all feel helpless as hell. So we cook to fight death, the enemy, or at least go through the mindless, physical act of putting together something to eat.

In Genesis 25, Jacob made a pot of lentil soup to comfort his father, Isaac. Isaac was feeling off his game and off his feed, having just buried his own father, Abraham (who made it to 175, if you can believe the Bible). Then Esau, Jacob's brother, comes in from the field and says, "Please let me have a swallow of that red stuff there, for I am famished." Jacob says not so fast, bro, I want your birthright, because according to scripture, Esau, the eldest male, was due to inherit everything. Esau is so hungry he thinks he's dying. He also thinks, what good is a birthright to a dead guy? So, fine, Jacob, here you go, hand over the soup.

Esau eats. He lives. He regrets. He hates his brother, he hates himself, and everyone loses. It is one of the earliest recorded histories of families behaving badly at a time of death and crisis.

That tradition endures. But so does the folk tradition of funeral food, the food you bring to the grieving. Over the centuries, the lentil has given way to food no one from Genesis would recognize, a parade of casseroles, spiral hams, deli platters, jiggling bowls of rice pudding, and dense funeral cakes. This is known in my family as DPF (dead people's food). It is food often absent of vegetables, though not absent of heart.

It is the heart, the caring I focus on when I'm red eyed and ragged out from crying and desperate for something green. I focus on how food lets us connect when all else fails. It is a bridge, the lingua franca of grief.

Patrick, too, was interested in what food can do, in a lab-experiment kind of way. Like if you take banana bread out of the oven now, when it needs to bake another forty minutes, walk it over to your next-door neighbor's oven, and finish baking it there, how will it come out? Pretty well, by the way.

Patrick loved process, and process happens at its own pace. He'd take an hour to make a salad. By the time it was ready, cocktails had gone on way too long; the lettuce had gone limp, and so had I.

Somehow, toward the end of his days, he'd made a lamb stew, which he froze in convenient if not biodegradable individual plastic containers. Marc found them after his death. He tried to throw them out. He couldn't.

Over a period of months, Marc heated them up and ate them. Patrick must have known he would. I bet Patrick, an altar boy gone astray, thought of this as a sort of communion, his way of having dinner with Marc even without being there in the flesh, a way of comforting his partner beyond the grave.

It's part of our human hardwiring to feed those who mourn. It is not a matter of addressing hunger; it is about coaxing and calling the grieving back into the riot of joy and pain and beauty and chaos that is life. Even when you're not ready. To eat is to engage, to strengthen, to unwrap from that first layer of sorrow's embrace and partake of life force.

Listen. The world is knocking on your door. It's saying, let us in. We've brought food.

Red Lentil Soup with Indian Spices

This lentil soup is not the one that scotched Jacob and Esau's biblical brotherly love. It is safe to eat and will sustain and support the sad or sick. Rather than your basic brown lentils, which are serviceable but drab, this recipe uses red lentils. They cook in minutes and with the tomatoes give the soup a rosy, hopeful tint. The spicing is gentle and reminds you things will not always be so hard. The greens add signs of life, not to mention calcium, vitamin C, and tryptophan, the amino acid that promotes a sense of well-being. Can't have too much of that, especially now.

Serves 6

2 tablespoons olive oil
1½ teaspoons ground cumin
1 teaspoon ground coriander
½ teaspoon turmeric
Pinch of red pepper flakes
2 large onions, chopped
6 cloves garlic, minced
1 thumb-size piece fresh ginger, minced
1½ cups red lentils
5 cups Stone Soup (see page 84) or other vegetable broth
One 28-ounce can diced tomatoes
Juice of 1 lemon
2 handfuls fresh spinach or kale, chopped — add another
     handful if you're a greens freak like me
1 bunch fresh cilantro, chopped
Sea salt and freshly ground pepper

In a generous-size soup pot, heat the oil over medium heat. Add the cumin, coriander, turmeric, and red pepper flakes. Cook, stirring often, until the oil darkens and the spices turn fragrant, about 1 minute. Add the onions, garlic, and ginger, and cook, stirring occasionally, until the onions soften and turn translucent, a few minutes.

Add the lentils and cook, stirring, for a few minutes more, until the lentils deepen in color and glisten with the spiced oil.

Add the broth and the tomatoes and their juice, and bring to a boil. Cover, reduce the heat to medium, and simmer until the lentils are tender and have become one with the soup, about 30 minutes. Stir in the lemon juice.

If you want the soup to be silky and smooth, you may puree with an immersion blender, but really, it's not necessary. Jacob didn't. The lentils are small and soft and have coalesced into the soup.

Gently stir in the spinach and cilantro. They will wilt into the soup. Season with salt and pepper.

The soup keeps several days in the fridge.

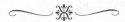

I get that death is humankind's own sort of renewal — out with the old lot, in with the new. Still, I think the process is flawed, and can't believe no one's come up with a better way.

I missed Patrick. I still miss him, but something strange happened. The terrible ache for him gave way to life, to people bearing food, and to Patrick himself. Being dead was no impediment; he just nudged it aside. He moved through me, he moved into me. He haunts me in pleasing ways. When I tell a funny story and people laugh, I know it's because of Patrick, and I know he's laughing, too. I can smell his coffee breath. He hasn't supplanted who I am — I will always be nervous. But he has become the best parts of me.

The ghosts I hang out with were wonderful to me in life. They're still good company, even dead. We talk to each other. It doesn't take a séance; it just takes me in the kitchen. Olives, capers, anything salty brings David, my father-in-law. Cookies conjure Marcella, who loved to bake them, and Patrick, who loved to eat them and was forever brushing sugar out of his beard.

Maybe your ghosts can be bought off with food offerings and such; mine tend to stick around, especially Marcella and Patrick. They still love a party.

I look around our Thanksgiving table, and the ghosts are there, really no different than they were in life — Patrick is saying outrageous things out of the corner of his mouth, just loud enough to make Marcella snigger and swat his arm. My grandfather Aaron harrumphs and cadges bits of turkey from the platter; my mother-in-law, uneasy, lips pressed, pushes food around on her plate as though it were suspect. David eats quickly, waiting till he and his second wife, the love of his life, can, politely, leave. She, slender, eats as though she hadn't in days, blinking and beaming, utterly amazed by the food. "I've never had this before. What do you call this? Stuffing? It's superb." All of them are dead. How is that possible?

There are new faces at the table, new friends, along with family like our niece Nikki, and beneath the table, our dog lies by our feet, praying for a morsel to drop. As the people we love become ghosts one by one, it seems there is less laughter at our holiday table but, perhaps, more tenderness. We, or at least I, recognize that even though we sometimes annoy the hell out of each other, our time together is precious. Finite. And we don't want to blow it.

Turkey I could do without, but I have a soft spot for Thanksgiving, where the food traditions come from your culture, your family. The corn-bread dressing my mother and I make together has its origins in the corn-bread dressing she used to make with Marcella. Over the years, we've added more vegetables to the dressing and enlisted the aid of a food processor.

I'm the heretic who put new twists on family favorites. I've introduced kale to our Thanksgiving table and enlisted Nikki to add the walnuts at the end. That is her holiday role. As she gets older, I'll have other things in store, to make her feel invested, to show Thanksgiving depends on her.

It depends on all of us. It's about remembering all we have and about remembering each other; it's about celebrating with the foods of the season. It's about getting together whether we feel like it or not, so we get a remedial lesson in our tribal ways. I suppose some people feel this way about the Super Bowl.

Thanksgiving Kale with Fennel, Cranberries, and Walnuts

This dish can be made a day ahead and can be served hot or at room temperature. It's easy, it's a gem, and cranberries add their own gemlike glam factor.

Serves 6 to 8

2 tablespoons olive oil
1 fennel bulb, cut into bite-size cubes
2 big bunches kale, chopped
¼ cup sherry
Pinch of red pepper flakes
⅓ cup dried cranberries
⅓ cup walnuts
Sea salt and freshly ground pepper

In a large pot, heat the oil over medium-high heat. Add the fennel to the pot. Cook, stirring occasionally, until softened, about 10 minutes.

Add the kale, a handful at a time, and cook until it just wilts but is still bright green, about 8 minutes. Stir in the sherry, red pepper flakes, and cranberries. Remove from the heat. (The kale mixture can be stored in an airtight container in the refrigerator for a day; bring to room temperature before proceeding with the recipe.)

Preheat the oven to 350°F.

Pour the walnuts into a shallow ovenproof pan and toast until they just turn golden brown and are fragrant, about 10 minutes. Remove from the oven and chop coarsely.

Gently reheat the kale in a large pot over medium heat until heated through, about 8 minutes. Get a friend or family member to stir in the walnuts with love. Season with salt and pepper.

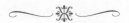

GENTLE NUDGE *the* ELEVENTH: SLOW FOOD

Sitting down to a meal has always been a way to celebrate. It says nourishment, it says abundance, it says delicious. And it shouldn't be reserved for Thanksgiving or Christmas; you can do it for a simple meal of soup tonight and get the same thrill. It may be the only part of your day when you relax.

Relaxing does not come naturally to me. I am much better at hunching my shoulders and clenching my jaw. But relaxing is as important to health as a workout, so I sit down, unlock my jaw, breathe deeply, and eat. It's better for digestion and ups the odds I'll actually taste my food. Eating at my desk or having a "working lunch" with colleagues leaves my brain and stomach feeling like the victims of a drive-by.

Factor in a little time in your day to do the same, to let go, to breathe, to slow down and eat. If you don't, you'll wind up producing quarts of cortisol. This is the fight-or-flight hormone your adrenal system pumps out in crisis mode. In a calamity situation, cortisol is what you want. It speeds up your response time and your heart rate. As a regular diet, however, cortisol drives up your blood pressure, increases your risk of heart attack, winnows your bone density and muscle mass, and — here's the especially charming bit — increases abdominal fat. Um, thanks, no.

Slowing down dials down the cortisol. It also ramps up the mindfulness, which is excellent in the grand scheme of things, leading to enlightenment, serenity, and all that. It also increases sensuality, which makes everything more fun right now.

Really. Stick out your arm. Excellent. Bring it back to your side. Now, take five whole seconds to raise it again. You may have more suppleness in your arm this time, rather than keeping it stick straight, as before. Observe the beauty in the languorous movement, feel the way your breath becomes deeper and more rhythmic. It's the same action as before, seasoned with just a little time. And appreciation. And sensuality. As James Baldwin wrote, "To be sensual, I think, is to respect and rejoice in the force of life, of life itself, and to be *present* in all that one does, from the effort of loving to the breaking of bread. It will be a great day for America, incidentally, when we begin to eat bread again, instead of the blasphemous and tasteless foam rubber that we have substituted for it." Well, that seems to call for a bread recipe, does it not?

No-Knead Whole Wheat Oatmeal Bread

Healthful and homemade, this is about the easiest yeast bread going. It gets its grainy goodness from whole wheat flour and oatmeal and needs no kneading. That's right. As with many no-knead bread recipes, this one owes its origins to Jim Lahey, mad genius bread baker and owner of New York's Sullivan Street Bakery.

Makes 1 loaf

One ¼-ounce packet active dry yeast
2 cups lukewarm water
1 tablespoon molasses
4 cups whole wheat flour
1 tablespoon olive or canola oil
¾ cup old-fashioned oats (also known as rolled oats)
¼ teaspoon sea salt

Pour the yeast into a large bowl. Add the warm water and molasses, and stir gently until the yeast dissolves. Let the yeast proof on your kitchen counter or a similar warm environment for 10 to 15 minutes.

When the yeast is frothy, add the flour. Mix well by hand, or with a mixer on low speed for 2 to 3 minutes, creating a smooth, moist, not sticky dough. Using a big spoon, work in the oil, oats, and salt until the dough just comes together. Do not obsess or overmix. Less is more.

Cover the bowl with a kitchen towel. Set in a warm spot to rise until doubled in bulk, about 1 hour. Lightly oil a 9-x-5-inch loaf pan or a 9-inch pie pan.

Punch down gently to let a bit of the air out. Do not pummel. Plop the dough into the prepared loaf pan or shape into a round and place in the pie pan.

Cover with the kitchen towel again and let the dough rise in a warm spot for 1 hour more. It should impress you by doubling again in size.

Preheat the oven to 450°F.

Bake for 30 minutes, or until the top is golden brown and crusty and the bread sounds hollow when tapped.

Well wrapped and refrigerated, it keeps several days. Warm up in the oven for a few minutes for maximum enjoyment.

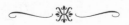

So there, you have sensuality and a lovely loaf of home-baked bread, too.

From preparing it to eating it, food is like foreplay, a pleasure in and of itself, one you don't want to rush. Allow yourself to get in the mood. Then sit down and enjoy your dinner. Enjoy yourself. You're a great date. Have fun. You owe it to yourself and to the planet to be happy.

That loaf of bread will be all the more delicious when paired with soup, particularly Tuscan White Beans and Winter Greens Soup.

Tuscan White Beans and Winter Greens Soup

Beans and greens again, but the flavor and body are very different than with the red lentil soup. And you make it with water — not vegetable broth, not stone soup. Water. I owe it — and much gratitude — to Italian culinary goddess Lidia Bastianich, from whom this recipe is adapted. It gets its goodness and oomph from the beans' own cooking liquid. Half a dozen sage leaves impart an amazing amount of flavor. It's just the thing for cool weather, costs a few bucks all told, and feeds six. And you'll have done it yourself. Beans may be cooked a day ahead, if that reduces your anxiety. Plan your life accordingly. Sit down and eat. Slowly.

Serves 6

1 pound dried white beans (cannellini, great Northern —
    whatever moves you)
4 tablespoons olive oil
5 cloves garlic
6 fresh sage leaves

2 dried red peppers
1 bay leaf
1 small head escarole or kale, finely chopped
1 cup white wine
Sea salt and freshly ground pepper

Place the beans in a large soup pot with a tight-fitting lid. Add enough water to cover the beans by 1 inch. Add 3 tablespoons of the olive oil, 4 garlic cloves, the sage, 1 dried red pepper, and the bay leaf. Bring to a boil over high heat.

Cover, reduce the heat to low, and simmer unattended for 90 minutes. Check your e-mail, have a quickie, watch *Mad Men*, whatever.

Check the beans; they should be soft, tender, and rich with flavor from the sage and garlic. Fish out the sage, the bay leaf, and the dried red pepper. (The beans can be stored in an airtight container in the refrigerator for a day; reheat the beans in a soup pot over medium-high heat before proceeding with the recipe.)

In a large skillet, heat the remaining 1 tablespoon of oil over medium-high heat. Mince the remaining garlic clove. Add the minced garlic, the remaining dried red pepper, and the escarole, a handful at a time, to the skillet. Cook until the escarole just wilts but is still a pretty celadon green, about 3 minutes.

Pour ½ cup of the wine into your pot of beans. Using a wooden spoon or an immersion blender, smash the beans until they turn creamy. Go as smooth as you like — I like to leave some beans whole for a nice rustic feel. Heat over medium-high heat until heated through, stirring occasionally

Stir in the wilted greens and the remaining ½ cup wine. Cover, reduce the heat to low, and continue cooking until the flavors mellow and blend, about 15 minutes. If the mixture seems too thick, add an additional ½ cup water. Season generously, because you're generous of heart, with salt and pepper.

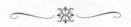

SWEETNESS *and* LIGHT

In the West, when we think of the winter holidays, we think of Christmas, with houses and fir trees bedecked with strands of pretty, winky lights. We think of Hanukkah, also known as the Festival of Lights, when we light candles in a menorah, a candelabra of sorts. But you know, the Judeo-Christian holidays of winter don't have a lock on light.

Kwanzaa has its own menorah, only it's called a kinara. It's lit with seven candles — *mishumaa saba* — representing the holiday's seven core values, which include purpose and faith. Beginning the day after Christmas, this weeklong holiday marks a still point in the midst of winter's gift-giving frenzy. It's a new holiday — created only in the 1960s — paying tribute to who we are and where we came from. Like Thanksgiving, Kwanzaa is secular, a centering celebration of culture, a handing down of ethnic principles and customs and foods, the things that shape society.

I wish there were a whole holiday dedicated to broccoli. Kwanzaa, at least, comes close. It means "first fruits of the harvest," and one of the holiday's symbols is *maʒao* — crops.

African American Sweet Potato and Peanut Stew

This stew contains peanuts, sweet potatoes, and black-eyed peas, a nutrient-dense triumvirate to warm you in winter. Serve over brown rice or millet, an ancient whole grain gift from Africa.

Serves 4 to 6

2 tablespoons canola or coconut oil
1 onion, chopped

1 jalapeño chili, minced, or a generous pinch of red pepper
   flakes
2 stalks celery, chopped
1 sweet potato, chopped
1 pound green beans, trimmed and halved
1 red bell pepper, chopped
1 cinnamon stick
2 cups cooked black-eyed peas (see Hopping John recipe,
   page 16) or one 15-ounce can black-eyed peas, rinsed
   and drained
One 15-ounce can diced tomatoes
2 tablespoons peanut butter
Sea salt and freshly ground pepper
1 handful fresh cilantro, chopped

In a large soup pot, heat the oil over medium-high heat. Add the
onion and jalapeño and cook for 1 minute. Add the celery, sweet
potato, green beans, and red bell pepper. Cook, stirring occasionally,
until the vegetables soften, a few minutes. Add the cinnamon, the
black-eyed peas, and the tomatoes and their juice. Cover, reduce the
heat to low, and simmer, stirring occasionally, until the stew thickens and the flavors develop, about 30 minutes.

Gently stir in the peanut butter until it dissolves and becomes
one with the stew. Season with salt and pepper. Gently stir in the
cilantro.

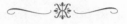

Lyon's Fête des Lumières — Festival of Lights — dates back to
1643, when the plague hit. Doesn't sound like fun. The townspeo-
ple agreed every home would light a candle for the Virgin Mary
and set it in the window, in hopes the plague would spare their

town. It worked. The city erected the Basilica of Notre-Dame de Fourvière in 1872 to honor the Virgin Mary and now marks December 8 as a day of gratitude, remembrance, and light. The whole town is set aglow, with high-tech light shows dressing up public spaces and candles lighting up every home.

Elsewhere in Europe, they celebrate St. Lucia's Day, named for a fourth-century Sicilian martyr who was said to consort with Satan. But that was probably a smear campaign to defame her. St. Lucia got in trouble for feeding persecuted Christians. She smuggled food to them at night, and so she could find her way hands-free, she designed the prototype of the helmet light. She wore a candelabra on her head. *Lucia* comes from the Latin word *lux*, meaning "light."

They still love her in Sicily, where they observe her feast day with bonfires, but she's really big in Sweden. On her feast day, December 13, which coincides with the winter solstice, young girls dress in white robes with red sashes and wear wreaths with candles on their heads. As a child, I was entranced by this. I also wondered, how do you not set your hair on fire?

In India, Diwali, the Hindu festival of lights, is observed by lighting candles and oil lamps and ends in a show of dazzling fireworks. The holiday has several backstories, but they all involve the destruction of some demon or other. It celebrates the triumph of good over evil, light over darkness. Like Kwanzaa, Diwali is about connection. It's a time when Indians contemplate and honor their relationship to others — friends, family — but also their relationship to the world and all the creatures in it.

At Diwali, Hindus rededicate themselves to living one of Hinduism's key precepts — *ahimsa*. We often translate it as "nonviolence" or "doing no harm." But it's not a negative; it's a positive — it's recognizing the sacredness in all of us. It's an ancient concept; the word itself comes from the Sanskrit. If we do it right, we get *samadhi* — divine, universal love.

No, really. Yoga began as a Hindu philosophy. It has eight limbs, all of which take you toward a higher state of being. Each of the limbs has its own components. Great idea, but way too many limbs. I was getting tangled up in the names and steps and legs and arms. It felt like playing a spiritual game of Twister against some hydra-headed creature, and I was going down.

Don't worry, a Hindu friend explained. It all starts with ahimsa. When you predicate everything you do on love, from the way you look at people to the way you eat, the other limbs seem to radiate out from there. He calls what we practice here Western yoga (and he's not quite ahimsa in the way he says it). What he means is, we learn a nifty crow pose, we learn *pranayama*, breathing control, where we snort through alternate nostrils. It seems pretty fab to us, but that's just the beginner level. Oh. So maybe that's why I've been practicing yoga for years now and have yet to find that whole surrender/serenity thing. The snorty business doesn't do much for me, either.

I'm more in tune with the Hindus when it comes to food and spirituality. They believe the two are intertwined. Food is sacred. Often it is first offered to the gods before we can eat it. This is called *prasadam* — God's mercy. That's why we must treat food with love and respect and humility, from growing the rice to cooking it. Remember chi? It's life force, it's energy. The chi we put into food infuses the food itself.

"If you bake bread with indifference, you bake a bitter bread that feeds but half man's hunger. / And if you grudge the crushing of the grapes, your grudge distils a poison in the wine." That's not Mario Batali talking; it's Kahlil Gibran. Just how talented the poet was in the kitchen is unknown, but I can vouch for what he wrote.

When I'm troubled, my spirit, apparently believing misery loves company, sabotages anything I attempt in the kitchen. My vinaigrette will erode the tender skin of your upper palate, nor will it do much for the salad greens. The quinoa will clump, and the muffins will be mush. You might want to pick up dinner somewhere else.

Love, on the other hand, transforms even the simplest dish. It makes our inner light shine, as with your basic yogic greeting — *namaste*, which means "I honor the light in you; you honor the light in me."

Diwali is based on the Hindu calendar and falls somewhere between late October and mid-December. It honors the harvest. At least on paper. Say "Diwali" to my Hindu friend, and he breaks into a megawatt grin suitable for the festival of lights. He isn't thinking of ahimsa; he's hungry for Diwali mithai, jewellike Indian sweets of semolina, nuts, fruit, warming spices, and sugar. And more sugar. Sitting in sugar syrup.

Diwali is about light, but it's also about sweets. All the winter holidays are.

On St. Lucia's Day, the girls of Sweden play St. Lucia herself by serving their families coffee and sweet spice buns known as lussekatter — Lucy cakes. How do they do this wearing flammable headgear? What do they do about hot, dripping wax? They're supposed to resemble the martyred St. Lucia, not become her.

There can be a degree of martyrdom involved with making the favorite sweet at Hanukkah, sufganiyot — little yeast-dough puffs fried in oil. They're akin to Greek loukoumades, Russian ponchiki, or Spanish bunuelos. The official story is they honor the original Hanukkah miracle — the light in the temple that somehow burned for eight days on a day's worth of oil. The truth of it is, people love fried food, and any excuse is good. The other truth is, frying adds calories and fat but no nutrients to your meal. My own personal truth is I'm fry averse and find dealing with hot, splattering oil almost as death defying as wearing candles on your head. Plus cleaning up afterward makes me cranky. Crankiness defeats the purpose.

Christmas sweets — where to begin? Candy canes, gingerbread men, yule-log Christmas cakes, a bazillion versions of Christmas cookies, and, of course, the ever-contentious fruitcake.

I will out myself. I love fruitcake — the real stuff, with its origins not in a factory but in ancient Rome. Fruitcake dates back to the fifth century, appearing in *De re coquinaria* (*The Art of Cooking*), the oldest surviving cookbook in the Western world. Back in the day, your prototypical fruitcake comprised simple ingredients, mostly chopped dried fruits and nuts. Within simplicity can lie complexity. The sumptuous oils of pine nuts, walnuts, almonds, and pistachios embraced and enhanced the winey sweetness of dates, apricots, plums, and raisins for a rich confection that endured (without preservatives) long after Rome fell.

It is the great-grandmother of sugarplums, the traditional English sweetmeats. All dried fruit were plums as far as the Brits of the Middle Ages were concerned. The sugarplums that danced in their heads were confections of nuts and dried fruit their ancient forebears might recognize.

And here we are today, with much of what we eat made of ingredients unrecognizable by ourselves. Do we eat too much processed food? Yes. Too much processed sugar? Yes. But sweetness is there for a reason. Some food historians believe we gravitate toward sweet food because in ancient agrarian times, when food was scarce, we turned to nutrient-rich dates and honey to sustain us. Good story.

I think we want to get it right. We want to be good and loving; we want to be sweetness and light. We just need some incentive. Honey, cookies, candy, yule logs, and sugarplums sweeten our mouths and our spirits. Sweetness primes the pump; it encourages us to be good. We are all, at heart, tantrumy two-year-olds. Bribe us with a cookie, and maybe we'll behave. The winter holidays have their backstories — the whole birth-of-Christ thing for Christmas and the rededication of the temple for Hanukkah — and here is where it gets tricky and divisive. Strip away the details, and the message is the same — miracles are possible, be it a star that lights up the night or the temple light that keeps burning when it should have gone out. We will care for the persecuted and vanquish the baddies. Including our own. We have both goodness and evil within us, and triumphing over our own dark impulses is the real miracle.

Hey, don't you religious guys even talk to each other? We could have one big holiday, all of us. We may belong to different faiths, different clubs, but we're more alike than we are different. Handily enough, Kwanzaa celebrates *umoja*, community.

If it's a matter of finding the common element, look no further than dessert. Sweetness has been part of our culture — all our cultures — for millennia. It's a far more effective way to reinforce what all these holidays teach us than the commercial buying fest we engage in these days. Toys and gadgets break. Often on Christmas morning. What endures are *samadhi* and *umoja*. You may not have known the words before, but you know what they mean.

Multifaith Sweetness and Light Sugarplums

These sugarplums require no cooking, no fuss, no frying, no candelabra. They get their sweetness naturally, from dates, common in many Middle Eastern desserts. Cardamom is beloved in both India and Sweden. The religions may view things differently, but we all share a desire for sweetness and light. File this under things you can throw together in a food processor that come out quite good.

Makes 2 dozen sugarplums

12 dried Medjool dates, pitted
8 dried apricots
½ teaspoon cardamon seeds
½ teaspoon anise seeds
1½ cups walnuts
¼ cup ground cinnamon or unsweetened cocoa powder

Put the dates and apricots in a food processor and pulse briefly, until they form bits that just start to come together in a mosaic. Add the cardamom seeds, anise seeds, and walnuts. Pulse again until just combined; the mixture will not quite adhere to itself. For lack of a better word, we can call it dough.

Wrap and chill the dough for at least 2 hours and up to overnight.

Pour the cinnamon (or cocoa) into a shallow bowl. Grab a generous pinch of the dough and roll into a ball about the size of a walnut. Roll the dough ball in the cinnamon until it's dusted on all sides. Continue with the remaining dough until you have 2 dozen sugarplums. The dough tends to absorb the spice, so roll the balls in the cinnamon a second time; they'll be prettier, more uniform, and easier to handle.

The sugarplums can be stored in an airtight container in the refrigerator for 2 weeks or more; the flavor improves over time.

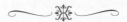

GENTLE NUDGE *the* PENULTIMATE: YOUR DAILY SERVING *of* AHIMSA

If you thought meditation was challenging, ahimsa will challenge you at a whole new level. It means doing no harm to a single creature, whether it's the ant you inadvertently flatten on your way out the door or your boss. Oh, you wouldn't really hurt your boss, of course. Not physically. Not intentionally. But the ratty, mean, low-down thoughts you — or at least I — have a dozen times a day are anti-ahimsa, too. Negative energy counts.

Ahimsa is not the same as sit-on-your-ass passivity. When supreme love guides everything you do, it is actually the ultimate power. At least that's the theory. Perfect ahimsa is not possible because we're not made perfect. No sense going around trying to act more ahimsa than thou. All we can do is practice ahimsa with humility and strive to get it more right than wrong most days.

How does it feel to come at the world from a loving place? Relaxing. Your shoulders are down, your face relaxed; your chest — and heart — feel open. You can let the world in and your love out. It feels like chai tastes — warm with spice, sweet, and creamy. It feels pleasantly evolved.

If you're having a crappy day, you might want a cup of chai to help you get there. When you're feeling more loving, you have more love to give.

Also known as masala tea, this Indian blend of black tea and sweet seasonings boosts serenity, circulation, and good spirits. In Indian restaurants, it's usually served with steamed milk, like a latte. A version of chai may be served in your favorite café or coffee shop, often with a whole lot of added sugar. I make it unsweetened and with almond milk, which complements the spices and has a richer mouth feel than soy. But use vanilla soy if you prefer, and sweeten as you wish. Think of chai as eggnog without the egg and booze but with all the spice and happy-making qualities intact. Unlike eggnog, it's served hot, all the more warming and welcoming in winter.

Ahimsa Chai

Serves 4 to 6

1 smallish lump of fresh ginger, minced
½ teaspoon cardamom seeds
1 cinnamon stick
4 whole cloves
½ teaspoon anise seeds
A few peppercorns
4 cups water
A full infuser of loose black tea or 4 black tea bags (may be decaffeinated)
1 cup almond milk or vanilla soy milk

Drop the ginger, cardamom, cinnamon, cloves, anise, and peppercorns into a medium saucepan. Add the water and bring to a boil

over high heat. Cover, reduce the heat to low, and simmer for
10 minutes. Uncover the saucepan and drop in the tea infuser. Re-cover
the saucepan and simmer, letting the tea steep, for about 5 minutes.

In a small saucepan, heat the almond milk over medium-high
heat, until it just reaches a boil. Turn off the heat.

Strain the tea into mugs or teacups, adding as much steamed
almond milk as desired.

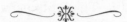

I do not automatically bound out of bed each morning feeling all
full of ahimsa. Being plant based at least offers a leg up. If a creature gave its life for your dinner, that not-ahimsa vibe is going to
catch up to you sometime. Going meatless has long been an integral part of Hindu practice. The Vedic text the Manusmriti or *The
Laws of Manu*, written sometime around 200 CE, argues the ethics
of eating meat back and forth, then concludes, "You can never
get meat without violence to creatures with the breath of life, and
the killing of creatures with the breath of life does not get you to
heaven; therefore you should not eat meat."

If the name of the text is almost impossible for a Westerner
to pronounce, the message is clear — a meatless diet promotes
ahimsa. It may even get you into heaven. Meanwhile, here on
earth, it encourages us to feel compassion toward everything with
the breath of life. That means all animals — including ourselves
and each other. Being meatless is healthful and holistic, leads to
a better integrated you, and racks up karmic goodness, too. At
the very least, it means we're not making things worse. And it's
anything but bland.

A meatless diet may be more than you're ready to bite off,
metaphorically speaking. Try doing it for one meal. For one day.
See where it takes you on life's journey.

Veggie Bhaji

Celebrate Diwali — or any day — with this vegetable bhaji. It's quick to make and fireworks-bright, with just a bit of jalapeño providing a small, pleasant explosion in the mouth. With a food processor fitted with the shredding disk, it's a breeze to make. Otherwise, seize your favorite chef's knife and slice the vegetables finely. It will go quickly. Think of the light. Purple cabbage adds eye appeal, fancier cabbage like napa or savoy is more tender and cooks quickly — the variety you use is your call.

Serve with brown basmati rice, or scoop up with naan, roti, or another flatbread (see Flatbread from a Starter, page 214).

Serves 4 to 6

3 tablespoons canola or coconut oil
1 tablespoon black mustard seeds
1 teaspoon ground cumin
1 teaspoon turmeric
1 tablespoon unsweetened dried coconut (optional but
    very nice)
1 onion
½ head of purple, napa, or savoy cabbage
3 carrots
1 red bell pepper, sliced into skinny strips
1 jalapeño chili, minced
Juice of 1 lemon
1 bunch fresh cilantro, chopped
Sea salt

Shred the onion, cabbage, and carrots.
    In a large skillet, heat the oil over high heat. Add the mustard

seeds. Cover with a lid and cook until the mustard seeds pop, about 1 minute. Uncover the skillet, reduce the heat to medium, and add the cumin, turmeric, and coconut (if using). Cook, stirring often, until the spices start to toast and the mixture becomes fragrant, about 1 minute.

Add the confetti of vegetables to the skillet and stir together over medium heat. Add the sliced red pepper and minced jalapeño to the skillet and cook, stirring occasionally, until the vegetables soften, about 10 minutes. Stir in the lemon juice and cilantro. Season with sea salt.

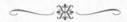

WHAT GOES AROUND COMES AROUND

As most American Jews, Muslims, Buddhists, Hindus, atheists, and Seventh-Day Adventists can tell you, Christmas in this country can make you feel like you're not in the club, like you're the Little Match Girl left out in the cold, pressing your nose to the window while everyone else is inside at a party where the food and wine are abundant, the home is warm and lovely, and everyone likes each other. That snow-frosted Christmas myth is so pervasive, we even try to pull it off in Miami, where it loses something in translation. Santas aren't supposed to sweat.

I was thrilled to marry into Benjamin's Lutheran family, thinking, ah, at last, I'll learn the secret Christmas handshake. What can I say? You were not there to warn me or say, "As if."

The Scots call the week between Christmas and New Year's Eve the Daft Days. The practice dates back to the Middle Ages, when it was created as a few days when you had license to be merry, cut loose, have a good time. We're still daft. But not always in a merry way. We reel from party to family gathering to command performance, half-mad from forced gifting and gaiety, fueled by guilt and an overabundance of the wrong sorts of things to eat and drink. All this merriness seems engineered to bring on a case of the low-downs in anyone less saintly than Tiny Tim.

One year, because Benjamin and I felt there weren't enough parties, not enough stress and togetherness and gift giving, we did the extradaft thing. We got married.

Often we celebrate our anniversary — and escape the rest of the daftness — by running away. If the airports are crowded, the timing is otherwise brilliant. No one works that week. Oh, they may show up at the office, but they're busy picking through what's left of the gift baskets and frantically placing gift orders online for people they'd forgotten about. You can go far during the Daft Days and will not much be missed.

When we can, we prefer out-of-the-country travel. Other cultures serve to remind us that not everyone associates Christmas with big, inflatable Santas, relentless piped-in carols, and maxed-out credit cards. It's our way of centering, our own reboot, a few days to set aside the daily distractions and focus on why we were daft enough to fall in love in the first place.

According to song and rumor, April in Paris is magical. I've only seen it in December. It's not half-bad then, either. If you're going to do the whole midnight-mass thing, Notre-Dame is the place to do it. High Gothic arches, booming organ, taking part with thousands of others in a rite dating back to the twelfth century — it all made me shiver with awe. I also shivered from the cold seeping up through the punishing stone floor. I kept shivering long afterward, as we walked back to our inn, in the cold and the pouring rain (Paris taxis stop running at midnight). So what? It was all part of the whole authentic experience.

This was followed by a few more authentic gray, rainy days and nights. Finally, the sun broke out — on our anniversary. The angels escaped from heaven, and the sky blossomed the rich shade known as French blue.

I stopped shivering and unbuttoned my coat as we walked through the bright streets of the Marais, slowed at a corner *fleuriste* to admire a profusion of tulips, turned to smile at Benjamin. He was gone.

I found him half a block back, leaning outside the door of a patisserie in a beam of sunlight. He had a blissed-out look on his face, a white paper sack in his hand — and something in his mouth. He kissed me with sugar-frosted lips.

"Éclair!" he announced, then licked his fingers.

This is one of the many things I love about Benjamin — his capacity for delight, his ability to treat himself right because he deserves it, his unswerving belief that you deserve it, too. He would have made a terrible Puritan, but if it's joy you're after, he's your man.

He led me to a restaurant at the Place des Vosges, and after a week of marvelous, memorable meals, I was in love before we'd even been seated. An array of towering white and butter-colored lilies welcomed us at the entrance, fresh, woodsy, with their slight scent of decay. Farther inside lay the proprietress's elderly dachshund, curled up in her basket on the floor. She raised her bearded muzzle as we walked by. She didn't wag her tail — how gauche, how American. But she regarded me through rheumy eyes with a certain *tendresse*, a sense of recognition, of ahh, I see you have come at last.

We were seated at a white-clothed table by the window. Sunlight spilled in and suffused us with gold.

Since it was a restaurant, there was also food, and if ever you had doubts as to what seasonal wonders winter offers, just remember truffles. The day's specials included salade aux truffes.

Well. Nine times out of ten, I'll take the cheap road. On the other hand, I'm not stupid. When great fortune kisses you on the lips and offers you black Périgord truffles, you don't smack it in the face. I ordered the priciest salad I have ever had in my life.

The softest of greens cupped a profusion of mushrooms — *champignons* in French, the word sounding tantalizingly like *champagne*. The salad was set off with thinly shaved radishes and roasted hazelnuts, dressed with the lightest sparkle of a genius French herb-lemon vinaigrette, and garnished with a generous shaving of Périgord truffles. They melted on the tongue, tasting of sun-filtered forest and something a little fuggy and naughty.

It was warm, wild, tender, chewy, gnarly, silky all at once. My heart raced. I scooped some salad onto a fork, aimed it at Benjamin's mouth. "You must taste this."

He took a bite, and the look of pleasure on his face doubled my own. Here I was in this wonderful place, with profligate flowers and proper dog, a gentle, smiling proprietress, in Paris, on a sunny day with my favorite person in the world. And truffles. I took a moment to do what Benjamin is much better at — I celebrated the moment. I gasped at my luck and grinned. If I looked like an idiot, just at that moment I did not care. Euphoria came off me like Chanel No. 5.

"We'll Always Have Paris" Wild Mushroom Salad

Perhaps you have to be French to master a perfectly balanced herb-and-lemon vinaigrette, but I hope this comes close. This salad aims to be like the one that inspired it, providing an exciting combination — warm, chewy, crispy mushrooms; cool, whisper-soft greens; round, hard nuts; crunchy disks of radish. Textures, temperatures, and flavors that all come together. In a Parisian sort of way.

Wild is wonderful, and winter is the season for rich, wild mushrooms. But, yes, you can throw a few tame white button mushrooms into the salad; all will be well.

Serves 2

¼ cup hazelnuts

1 tablespoon olive oil

1 clove garlic, minced

8 ounces assorted seasonal wild mushrooms, such as oyster
    mushrooms, cèpes, morels, hen-of-the-woods, wiped
    clean and sliced

3 big handfuls arugula, watercress, and/or tender lettuce
    leaves, like butter or red leaf lettuce

4 tablespoons hazelnut or walnut oil

3 tablespoons fresh lemon juice

1 tablespoon finely chopped fresh tarragon

Sea salt and freshly ground pepper

4 to 6 radishes, such as watermelon radishes or French
    Breakfast radishes, thinly sliced

A shaving of truffles, if you've got 'em

Truffle, hazelnut, or walnut oil for drizzling (optional)

Heat a large dry skillet over medium-high heat. Pour in the hazelnuts. Toast the nuts for about 7 minutes, shaking the skillet or chasing the hazelnuts around with a wooden spoon. They'll roll around in the skillet like marbles. When they begin to darken and smell unbelievably buttery and fragrant, pour the hazelnuts off into a small bowl and let cool.

No need to wipe out the skillet. Use it to heat the olive oil over medium-high heat. Add the garlic. Cook, stirring often, until the garlic softens and turns golden, 3 to 4 minutes. Add the mushrooms, in batches, if necessary. Allow enough space in the pan. We don't like to be crowded, neither do mushrooms — it will make them soggy.

Raise the heat to high. Cook, prodding mushrooms with a spatula. Keep them moving until they darken and smell rich and earthy, 4 to 5 minutes. Give the mushrooms a flip and continue cooking on the other side, for 4 to 5 minutes more. The secret to this dish is the texture — the mushrooms should be tender but with a crispy outside.

In the meantime, mound the arugula on two salad plates or a single serving platter.

In a small bowl, whisk together the hazelnut oil, lemon juice, tarragon, a pinch of sea salt, and a good grind of pepper.

Scatter the crisped mushroom slices over the arugula, fling the radishes around on top, and strew with hazelnuts.

Pour the dressing over all. Taste and season with salt and pepper, if desired.

Lovely.

If you want to be decadent like the Parisians, top with truffle shavings and drizzle with truffle oil.

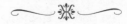

The couple at the table beside us inclined their heads toward me and smiled, then turned back to enjoying their meal, a bottle of

wine, and each other. Their voices were low, their laughter generous. Her gunmetal-gray dress fell in fabulous folds around her;
he wore a black sweater with a subtle gloss, as though woven by
silkworms who adored him.

The man turned back to us, gestured to the wine, and gave
us a radiant smile. "We aren't going to drink all this," he said in
impeccable, unaccented English. "Would you perhaps share some
with us?"

In Miami, strangers don't offer you wine. Or if they do, I fear
they've spiked it with drugs. But on this day in Paris, it seemed
like one more bit of magic we were being granted. We thanked
them, and the waiter brought two more glasses. The wine was, in
memory at least, a buttery Sauternes, warm and welcoming as the
sun, perfectly chilled so as not to shock the system or sensibili-
ties. It was a revelation. The first notes were musty, yeasty, flinty,
followed by the lovely pucker of dried apricots and fresh lemon.
Each sip told its own story.

The chic couple had a story, too. They were not from Paris
or even France, it turns out, but from Chicago. They came every
year. On their anniversary. Today was their thirtieth. Thirty
years? I recalculated their age. Maybe they were childhood sweet-
hearts. Even so, they were at least a decade older than I'd figured,
just in their early fifties, but I'm telling you, hot early fifties. Wow
— you could be older and still astonishingly sexy. This was as
exhilarating as the wine.

"What's your secret for a happy marriage?" I asked.

She smiled. "We believe in celebration."

It was clear to me we had to spend every minute with this
couple before we left Paris. And maybe move to Chicago when
we got home. Right next door to them.

I don't know why I'm wired this way, but I am. If I meet you and I like you, you're screwed because I'm going to want us to be best friends forever and to know everything about you *right now*, from what you ate for breakfast to who your favorite Karamazov brother is. Sometimes I think my avidity, the way I fall in love with a place or a person or a pet or a plant, is charming. The rest of the time, I just want to muzzle myself.

Lacking any ability to filter, I said something to the effect of, "So what are you guys planning for tonight, and can we come, too?"

The woman smiled again, a warm, open gift of a smile, as though I wasn't being a stalker weirdo at all. She didn't say, "Back off, bitch," or slap me with a restraining order. She said, "This has been such a beautiful lunch. Let's just enjoy it now."

It was true; now had a lot going for it. But I wanted more. I always do. I prefer not to think of myself as needy — just someone who has not yet mastered the Buddhist concept of detachment.

Attachment is one of Buddhism's big soul poisons, which once caused me to believe, despite their otherwise loving and mellow ways, Buddhists were just being hard-assed. Detachment? What's the point? We must love each other as fiercely as we can, not be "cool," as Ralph Waldo Emerson put it, "for it will all be one a hundred years hence."

Over time, I have come to realize detachment is not the same as not caring, not loving. Love all you want; it's no skin off Buddha's ass. On the other hand, you — *I* — still have to be aware of, accept, and roll with the constant impermanence of things, what Buddhists call *anicca*.

We can't be sure of anything a hundred years hence. We can't be sure of much. All we have is this moment. That said, I still choose to love people fiercely. I'm not made any other way.

The fabulous Chicago couple parted company with us on that wondrous afternoon in Paris. They kissed our cheeks in French fashion, melted into the crowd, and disappeared. But the day did not vanish with them. Though Benjamin and I shared no more than an hour and a glass of wine with them, it is still a fragrant memory, something warming in winter I can conjure with a mere mushroom.

Bring your finger to the bridge of your nose. Right there on the other side of the nasal bone is your amygdala, the almond-shaped part of the brain conveniently close to your center of smell. This part of the brain houses memory. It's like an iPod for recollection. It's not into analysis; it stores the whole sensory gestalt of things. It also plays a role in the way we process emotion.

There's the whole physiology behind what makes us hungry for more than dinner. It's the mystery, the romance of it that enchants me. I cook. I create. And I remember. A smell or taste can bring the richness of a past moment roaring back and infuse the present with sweetness, from the golden sunlight and Sauternes that wonderful day in Paris to the way the halvah Marcella gave me melted on my tongue when I was a girl. It's such a clever part of us that it makes all our design flaws a soupçon more tolerable. It also shows there's power and opportunity in everything we do.

Both the planet and you are miracles, superior in form and function to anything we mere mortals have dreamed up. Both maintain a complex series of operating systems and usually manage them so effortlessly, we don't even notice. Okay, one of us is much, much larger than the other, so much as to make you feel insignificant at times. Don't be fooled. You are madly significant. The fate of the whole world depends on you, including what you eat for dinner.

We are badly worn by what has become of our environment, our food system, ourselves. What nations and religions have done and are doing to each other could turn us all bitter, take us farther apart. So how can food be the answer?

So much unseen has gone into the meal before you, the seasons the planet spent producing it, be it grapes, truffles, and hazelnuts, or rice and beans. There's the labor and care of those who make the wine, forage for the truffles, and fuss over the vinaigrette, or harvest and dry the grains and legumes. There's the culture and place and faith and history infusing any dish. You bring unseen magic to each meal, too, by way of your own unique memories and emotions and associations. The simplest meal is in truth a deliciously collaborative effort, a mystery both divine and earthly.

When grown and prepared with love and shared with others, food feeds our hunger now, but more than that, it feeds who we can be. It lights a path to understanding, to overcoming the dark, hungry parts of ourselves. A single moment, a single taste, can flavor a whole life and feed a primal hunger — for love, connection, a sure if fleeting faith that for once, all is right with the world. The question is, why? I'm willing to say it's there for us to be grateful for all we have. Gratitude is the soul's Lipitor. It opens our hearts. It gives us faith. It gives us energy to go forward. A Buddhist prayer ends, "May we accept this food for the realization of the way of love and understanding." Food should always lead us to that. And to each other.

Here are lentils and millet and garlic and saffron and cumin, the foods that have sustained us since before the Bible. Here are kale and broccoli and vibrant field greens that bespeak life force. Here is crusty, yeasty flatbread, still warm from being turned out of its pan. Dip it in this olive oil that flows golden green and tastes of grass and pepper. Here are dates and mangoes and figs and pomegranates to dazzle you with their sweetness. I will pour you wine the color of pomegranates, grown from old, wise grapevines. I will pour you hot, pale tea, fragrant with flowers, to heal your heart and feed your searching soul. They are all too precious to savor alone; they must be shared.

This kind of food, this kind of feeding, is a benediction, a seed that can take root. Look — watch it grow and blossom even as you look, Janus-like, forward into a whole new year.

It is not within me to smile like Buddha or the Mona Lisa and say everything happens for a reason. But I have faith enough to be grateful for now, to know, as Wordsworth did, "That in this moment there is life and food / For future years. And so I dare to hope."

We're here and alive. We're still in the game. Everything is possible. So come to the table.

GENTLE NUDGE
the ULTIMATE:
PRACTICE BARAKA

You know I can't let you go without a good meal.
Cooking for people is an ancestral calling in my blood. Maybe
I'm working off some bad karma from a past life. It feels like
good karma to me, though. From Marcel, my genius friend and
his magical soupe joumou to the women in Marrakech, singing
as they worked, so many people have nourished me in so many
ways. Food is always the way I think of to repay them. That they
might prefer a gift card is something I only consider after the fact.

Whether it's inviting strangers to drink your wine or friends
to eat your food, the shared meal has defined hospitality in every
faith and culture I know. And yet these days we do it only rarely.
We are too busy, or too timid, or too stuck in our ways. We would
rather text — quicker, easier, no fuss, no muss. What we risk losing is the subtext — our glorious mess, our humanity. What is the
point of having people in your life if you can't cook with them,
feed them? If you can't eat and drink and talk and laugh together,
all crowded around the table?

Every meal — *any* meal, no matter how humble — can offer the opportunity for deeper connection, for a communion for people of every faith or of no particular faith at all. We begin when we begin, be it the first day of the new year according to the Gregorian calendar, the Julian calendar, or the lunar calendar or when we're hungry. We create celebration when we gather. We create plenty by being our most authentic selves.

The Hebrew word for "blessing" or "prayer" is *baruch*. In Arabic, it is *baraka*. In Morocco, it means the same, but baraka is also its own kind of blessing. It is showing gratitude for the food you have by sharing it. It is creating abundance. It is the power to multiply food. You don't have to be Jesus to do it, either. This kind of blessing, the law of increase, requires a practical magic, of making the most of what you have, even when it's very little. Some people, like Marcel, are born with this gift. However, it can be learned.

Fresh, local produce is vibrant in the mouth and easy on the wallet. Whole grains and dried beans keep in your pantry like money in the bank. They're cheap, comforting, nourishing, and, with clever application, feed a horde. Steaming a pot of couscous or barley causes the tender grains to swell and expand. You can keep resteaming so the grains fluff and seem to proliferate, feeding as many as are at your table. With a little creativity, a well-stocked larder, and a desire to feed those you love, you'll be sure no one goes hungry.

I am grateful and fortunate to know Paula Wolfert, goddess of Moroccan and Mediterranean food ways. She not only taught me about baraka; she exemplifies it. I hope to follow her gracious example with this recipe, adapted from hers in *The Food of Morocco*.

Many Moroccan lamb or chicken tagines include preserved

lemon and olives — a wonderful, haunting combination. Many recipes for vegetable couscous include a handful of raisins. Many vegetable couscous recipes — even the classic seven-vegetable couscous — also include lamb or chicken. But not preserved lemon and olives. This does not seem to me the least bit fair. Not only do lamb and chicken receive unique culinary treatment, but they greedily find their way into messing up an otherwise lovely plant-based dish. With this vegetable couscous, I have hoped to right a terrible wrong. I have left out the raisins. And lamb. And chicken.

Cheap, simple produce seasoned by a miserly amount of extravagant spice served over a mound of whole grains, this Moroccan dish employs some of the techniques of a tagine but is served over whole wheat couscous or barley. It is baraka itself.

Vegetable Couscous with Preserved Lemon and Olives

Chopping the vegetables into larger pieces in this recipe helps them maintain their integrity during slow cooking. The olives should be good, imported ones, be they Moroccan or Greek or French or Italian, such as oily kalamatas or mild green Picholine or a combination. Traditionally, they're enjoyed whole, not pitted. Break with tradition as you wish.

Serve with every bit of the luscious broth over whole wheat couscous or barley and pair with Flatbread from a Starter (page 214).

Serves 4 to 6. Recipe may be doubled, even tripled, depending on how many surprise guests you have. There will always be enough.

2 tablespoons olive oil
4 cloves garlic, coarsely chopped
1 large onion, coarsely chopped
4 carrots, coarsely chopped
4 stalks celery, coarsely chopped
1 red bell pepper, coarsely chopped
1 zucchini, coarsely chopped
1 tomato, coarsely chopped
2 cups cooked chickpeas or one 15-ounce can chickpeas,
    rinsed and drained
1 cinnamon stick
Pinch of saffron
½ teaspoon ground ginger
½ teaspoon turmeric
2 cups Stone Soup (see page 84) or other vegetable broth
    or water
1 cup whole wheat couscous or barley
1 preserved lemon, finely chopped*
⅓ cup olives
Sea salt and freshly ground pepper
1 bunch cilantro, chopped

In a large soup pot, heat the oil over medium heat. Add the garlic and onion. Cook, stirring occasionally, until the vegetables soften, a few minutes. Add the carrots, celery, red bell pepper, zucchini, tomato, chickpeas, cinnamon stick, saffron, ginger, turmeric, and broth. Stir to combine. Cover, reduce the heat to low, and simmer for 10 minutes.

Uncover the soup pot and continue cooking until the vegetables are tender and the sauce has thickened and reduced, about 20 minutes.

---

* Preserved lemons are available at Middle Eastern and gourmet markets.

Prepare the couscous or barley according to the package directions.

Stir the preserved lemon and olives into the pot with the vegetables and spices. Season with sea salt and pepper. Just before serving, stir in the cilantro.

Pour the couscous into the bottom of a tagine or into a large, shallow serving bowl. Form a well in the center. Fill with the vegetables and broth. Enjoy.

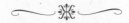

Breaking bread together is an ancient rite of welcome. It is also a revolutionary act. Ending all wars doesn't take another war. It takes a communal meal. We bring our traditions, our culture, and our core beliefs — the things we value — to the table. We may not agree, but we can sit together and talk about it over food. It is a way to bridge the differences between us, to meet all our hunger, to partake in baraka. It has been our best hope for humanity dating back to biblical days. In Acts 2:46, faith brought people together, but so did sharing food. "Every day they continued to meet together in the temple courts. They broke bread in their homes and ate together with glad and sincere hearts."

Here is bread to break. This is my go-to flatbread. Chewy and flavorful, it's not quite naan, nor true Moroccan bread, but it works very well with Veggie Bhaji (see recipe, page 197) or with the Vegetable Couscous with Preserved Lemon and Olives (see recipe, page 211) — with everything, really.

I adapted and veganized the recipe from one by the late, great food writer and novelist Laurie Colwin. "We *are* all brothers and sisters," as she wrote in "The Case of the Mysterious Flatbread." "This bread from Ethiopia is very similar to a bread from India or Scotland and is appreciatively devoured by a nice Jewish girl from Philadelphia, her husband, who was born in Latvia, and their New Yorker daughter." And, may I amend, further monkeyed with and even improved upon a by a passionate, spiritual, though secular vegan who passes it on to you as a means of increase and baraka. It's foolproof, forgiving, and fabulous — you will be very impressed with yourself.

Flatbread from a Starter

The flatbread starter takes just a few minutes to make. Then you leave it to its yeasty self to bubble and develop overnight. Making the bread dough takes only a few minutes more, and it needs only a couple hours to rise. You'll have to break the bread to share, but that's the whole point, isn't it? This flatbread is excellent served with Vegetable Couscous with Preserved Lemon and Olives (page 211), Veggie Bhaji (page 197), and any of the soups.

Serves 6 to 8

¼ cup unsweetened soy milk
1 tablespoon apple cider vinegar
1 teaspoon active dry yeast
1 cup plus 2 tablespoons warm water
1½ teaspoons evaporated cane sugar
2⅓ cups whole wheat flour, plus more as needed
½ teaspoon sea salt
Oil for the skillet

Pour the soy milk into a small cup or bowl. Add the vinegar. It will curdle; don't fret.

Pour the yeast into a medium bowl. Add 2 tablespoons warm water and the soy milk mixture.

Leave to froth for a few minutes.

Add the sugar and ⅓ cup of the flour. Stir together.

Cover the bowl with a kitchen towel and leave it on the counter or in a cool oven overnight.

The next afternoon, add 2 cups of the whole wheat flour, 1 cup warm water, and the sea salt to the starter.

Mix gently. Work in more flour, up to another ½ cup, until you have a sturdy, not sticky dough.

Cover the bowl with a kitchen towel again. Set in a warm spot to rise until doubled in bulk, 2 hours or longer.

Lightly oil an 8-inch skillet and heat over high heat.

Meanwhile, divide the dough into thirds. Flatten and stretch into rounds about 6 to 8 inches across, so that each piece of dough fits into the skillet.

Take one piece of dough and place on the skillet. Cook until tawny and pebbled with brown spots, 5 to 8 minutes per side. The flatbread is done when it's crusty and sounds hollow when tapped.

Repeat with the remaining balls of dough.

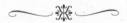

Maybe a time will come when the whole world can cook and eat together with glad and sincere hearts. Start by doing it with someone you know. Cook with your children. Ask a friend over for a meal. Make a kitchen date with your mother, your auntie, whoever's the keeper of the culinary flame, to learn how to make the dishes that bespeak home and celebration within your family. Host a potluck. Organize a block party. Invite everyone. There's always room for one more. We are stronger together than apart. Hungry ghosts and hungry people — we all love a party. So pull up a chair. Let's eat.

ACKNOWLEDGMENTS

A generous serving of gratitude to everyone who had faith that I could write this book and cheered me on all the way, often over a great meal, including:

Danielle Svetcov of Levine Greenberg
Georgia Hughes and all the fab folk at New World Library
Diana Abu-Jaber
Debra Dean and Cliff Fetters
Holly Gonzalez
Sharon Johnson
Lewis and Marcia Kanner
Tony Proscio and Peter Borrell
Jacqueline Rubens
Stefan Uch
Marc Zemsky

For their professional wisdom and unstinting good humor, I am grateful to:

Miami Herald food editor Kathy Martin
Culinate editor Kim Carlson
Mitchell Kaplan and Cristina Nosti of Books and Books
The staff of *Huffington Post*, most especially Green section editors Joanna Zelman, Travis Donovan, and Katherine Goldstein
Erica Meier and Jaya Bhumitra of Compassion Over Killing
Denise Ryan of the Organic Farming Research Foundation

In person, on the page, on the plate, the following people have carved out moments of grace in this often graceless age, and that is really what we're hungry for:

John Ash
Nava Atlas
Lidia Bastianich
Melissa Clark
Laurie Colwin
Mireille Giuliano
Gabrielle Hamilton
Michel Nischan
Michael Schwartz
Nigel Slater
Terry Theise
Paula Wolfert

For all of the above and more, thank you, Benjamin Bohlmann, wonderful husband, courageous accountant, outstanding traveling companion. You make my life delicious.

In putting together this list of acknowledgments, I am missing people. Please forgive — I owe you dinner.

NOTES

INTRODUCTION — HUNGRY ALL THE TIME

Page xiii, *glittering, rosy, moist, honied*: D. H. Lawrence, "Figs," Kalliope, accessed September 4, 2012, www.kalliope.org/en/digt.pl?longdid =lawrence2001061702.

Page xvii, *God's not all that interested*: Jaweed Kaleem, "Fallen Priest Alberto Cutie, Soon to Become a Dad, Rebuilds Miami Ministerial Life as an Episcopalian," *Miami Herald*, May 29, 2010.

CHAPTER 1: THE SEED

Page 23, *Walter de la Mare's poem*: Walter de la Mare, "Miss T.," in *Forget-Me-Nots: Poems to Learn by Heart*, ed. Mary Ann Hoberman (New York: Little Brown, 2012), 55.

Page 23, *Tell me what you eat*: Jean Anthelme Brillat-Savarin, *The Physiology of Taste; or, Meditations on Transcendental Gastronomy*, trans. M. F. K. Fisher (New York: Vintage Books, 2011), 15.

Page 23, *anybody to play with at all*: This and the following excerpts from "There Once Was a Puffin" are taken from Florence Page Jaques, "There Once Was a Puffin," in *The Harp and the Laurel Wreath: Poetry and Dictation for Classical Curriculum*, ed. Laura Berquist (San Francisco: Ignatius Press, 1999), 26.

Page 31, *what Oscar Wilde said*: Oscar Wilde, *The Importance of Being Earnest: A Trivial Comedy for Serious People*, act 2, Project Gutenberg, last modified August 29, 2006, www.gutenberg.org/files/844/844-h/844-h.htm.

Page 32, *University of North Carolina study*: Deborah F. Tate et al., "Replacing Caloric Beverages with Water or Diet Beverages for Weight Loss in Adults: Main Results of the Choose Healthy Options Consciously Everyday (CHOICE) Randomized Clinical Trial," *American Journal of Clinical Nutrition* 95, no. 3 (2012): 555–63, doi: 10.3945/ajcn.111.026278.

CHAPTER 2: THE FLOWERING

Page 51, *as Alfred, Lord Tennyson wrote*: Alfred, Lord Tennyson, "Locksley Hall," Poetry Foundation, accessed September 4, 2012, www.poetry foundation.org/poem/174629.

Page 55, *what James Joyce described*: James Joyce, *Ulysses* (New York: Random House, 1961), 55.

Page 66, *Behold, I have given you*: Bible, Genesis 1:29, English Standard Version.

Page 67, *Every moving thing*: Bible, Genesis 9:3, King James Version.

Page 67, *The weak person eats*: Bible, Romans 14:2, English Standard Version.

Page 67, *Let not the one who eats*: Bible, Romans 14:3, English Standard Version.

Page 68, *Meat commendeth us not*: Bible, 1 Corinthians 8:8, King James Version.

Page 68, *Better is a dinner*: Bible, Proverbs 15:17, English Standard Version.

CHAPTER 3: THE HARVEST

Page 105, *Summer surprised us*: T. S. Eliot, "The Waste Land," in *The Best Poems of the English Language: From Chaucer through Frost*, ed. Harold Bloom (New York: HarperCollins, 2004), 905.

Page 105, *The harvest is past*: Bible, Jeremiah 8:20, King James Version.

Page 110, *But ask the animals*: Bible, Job 12:7–10, New International Version.

Page 120, *Wordsworth wrote*: William Wordsworth, "The World Is Too Much with Us," in *The Complete Poetical Works of Wordsworth*, ed. Andrew J. George (Boston: Houghton Mifflin, 1932), 349.

Page 125, *Bowles's definition of magic*: Gena Dagal Caponi, *Conversations with Paul Bowles: Literary Conversations* (Jackson: University of Mississippi Press, 1993), 106.

CHAPTER 4: THE COMPOST

Page 168, *Millions of spiritual creatures*: John Milton, *Paradise Lost*, bk. 4, lines 677–78.

Page 182, *As James Baldwin wrote*: James Baldwin, "The Fire Next Time," in *The Price of the Ticket: Collected Nonfiction, 1948–1985*, p. 350, Google Books preview, accessed September 21, 2012, http://books.google.com/books ?isbn=0312643063.

Page 189, *If you bake bread*: Kahlil Gibran, "Work," in *The Prophet*, Wikilivres, last modified May 26, 2008, http://wikilivres.ca/wiki/The_Prophet/Work.

Page 196, *The Manusmriti*: Manusmriti 5:38.48.53, translated by Wendy Doniger, *The Hindus: An Alternative History* (New York: Penguin, 2009), 317.

Page 205, *as Ralph Waldo Emerson put it*: Ralph Waldo Emerson, "Montaigne; or, The Skeptic," in *Representative Men*, Ralph Waldo Emerson Texts, last modified September 3, 2009, www.emersoncentral.com/montaigne.htm.

Page 208, *as Wordsworth did*: William Wordsworth, "Lines Composed a Few Miles above Tintern Abbey," in *The Best Poems of the English Language: From Chaucer through Frost*, ed. Harold Bloom (New York: HarperCollins, 2004), 327.

EPILOGUE — GENTLE NUDGE THE ULTIMATE: PRACTICE BARAKA

Page 213, *Every day they continued*: Bible, Acts 2:46, New International Version.

Page 213, *We are all brothers and sisters*: Laurie Colwin, *More Home Cooking: A Writer Returns to the Kitchen* (New York: HarperCollins, 1993), 50.

DELICIOUS
RECOMMENDED
READING

Abu-Jaber, Diana. *The Language of Baklava*. New York: Anchor Books, 2006.

Allen, Will. *The Good Food Revolution: Growing Healthy Food, People, and Communities*. New York: Gotham Books, 2012.

Bittman, Mark. *How to Cook Everything Vegetarian: Simple Meatless Recipes for Great Food*. Hoboken, NJ: Wiley, 2007.

Brillat-Savarin, Jean Anthelme. Translated and edited by M. F. K. Fisher. *The Physiology of Taste; or, Meditations on Transcendental Gastronomy*. New York: Vintage Books, 2011.

Clark, Melissa. *Cook This Now: 120 Easy and Delectable Dishes You Can't Wait to Make*. New York: Hyperion, 2011.

Colwin, Laurie. *More Home Cooking: A Writer Returns to the Kitchen*. New York: HarperCollins, 1993.

Friese, Kurt Michael, Kraig Kraft, and Gary Paul Nabhan. *Chasing Chiles: Hot Spots along the Pepper Trail*. White River Junction, VT: Chelsea Green, 2011.

Hamilton, Gabrielle. *Blood, Bones & Butter: The Inadvertent Education of a Reluctant Chef*. New York: Random House, 2012.

Reichl, Ruth. *Tender at the Bone: Growing Up at the Table*. New York: Random House, 2010.

Slater, Nigel. *Toast: The Story of a Boy's Hunger*. New York: Gotham Books, 2005.

Theise, Terry. *Reading between the Wines*. Berkeley: University of California Press, 2011.

Van Aken, Norman, and Justin Van Aken. *My Key West Kitchen: Recipes and Stories*. London: Kyle Books, 2012.

Wolfert, Paula. *The Food of Morocco*. New York: Ecco, 2011.

INDEX

225

ABOUT *the* AUTHOR

Ellen Kanner is an award-winning food writer, Huffington Post's Meatless Monday blogger, and the syndicated columnist the Edgy Veggie. She is published in *Bon Appétit, Eating Well, Vegetarian Times, Every Day with Rachael Ray,* and *Culinate,* as well as in other online and print publications. She's an ardent advocate for sustainable, accessible food, serving on the Miami boards of Slow Food and Common Threads.

When she's not teaching underserved students to cook or speaking about what we're hungry for, Ellen takes time to tend her tiny organic vegetable garden, hike in the Everglades, make friends with cows, and make dinner with friends. There's always room for more at her table. She believes in close community, strong coffee, organic food, and red lipstick. A fourth-generation Floridian, she lives "*la vida* vegan" in Miami with her husband. Learn more about Ellen at www.ellen-ink.com.

NEW WORLD LIBRARY is dedicated to publishing books and other media that inspire and challenge us to improve the quality of our lives and the world.

We are a socially and environmentally aware company, and we strive to embody the ideals presented in our publications. We recognize that we have an ethical responsibility to our customers, our staff members, and our planet.

We serve our customers by creating the finest publications possible on personal growth, creativity, spirituality, wellness, and other areas of emerging importance. We serve New World Library employees with generous benefits, significant profit sharing, and constant encouragement to pursue their most expansive dreams.

As a member of the Green Press Initiative, we print an increasing number of books with soy-based ink on 100 percent postconsumer-waste recycled paper. Also, we power our offices with solar energy and contribute to nonprofit organizations working to make the world a better place for us all.

Our products are available
in bookstores everywhere.
For our catalog, please contact:

New World Library
14 Pamaron Way
Novato, California 94949

Phone: 415-884-2100 or 800-972-6657
Catalog requests: Ext. 50
Orders: Ext. 52
Fax: 415-884-2199
Email: escort@newworldlibrary.com

To subscribe to our electronic newsletter, visit
www.newworldlibrary.com

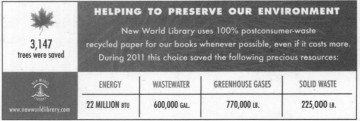

HELPING TO PRESERVE OUR ENVIRONMENT

New World Library uses 100% postconsumer-waste recycled paper for our books whenever possible, even if it costs more. During 2011 this choice saved the following precious resources:

3,147
trees were saved

www.newworldlibrary.com

ENERGY	WASTEWATER	GREENHOUSE GASES	SOLID WASTE
22 MILLION BTU	600,000 GAL.	770,000 LB.	225,000 LB.

Environmental impact estimates were made using the Environmental Defense Fund Paper Calculator @ www.papercalculator.org.